THE PERFECT SCALE

The Ultimate Fat Loss System

DOUG DORSEY

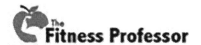

The information in this book is not intended as medical advice or to replace the services of trained health professionals. Be sure to consult with a health care professional before you implement any nutrition or exercise program.

ISBN: 978-0-9997756-0-8

www.TheFitnessProfessor.com

This book is dedicated to my mother

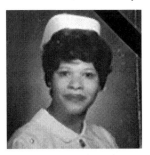

Winifred Rae Boyd
May 7, 1943 – November 13, 2017
Loving, sweet, intelligent, strong, fun and simple
Forever in my heart
#Winniesbabyboy

Contents

Acknowledgments

I want to thank all mighty God for my life, health, and strength. I am truly blessed and fortunate to serve in this capacity. Thank you for the Angels above that guide me.

I would like to express my gratitude to those who have supported and mentored me throughout my life. Writing a book has always been a life-long dream, and dreams only come true when you are surrounded by people looking out for your best interest. It was a long process, but WE made it. Thank you.

I would like to thank my family for your support and unconditional love. While they say you can choose your friends but you can't choose your family, I'd choose my family again and again and again.

I also want to thank my friends who have provided so much support, motivation, encouragement, and love during this entire process. Good friends are hard to find and I have the best. Kim, Karen, Bryan, and Steve, thank you for listening, asking how it's going, and encouraging me throughout the process.

Thank you to the entire crew that helped me put this book together. Self-publishing school, Coach—Scott Allan, Editor—Katie Chambers, Guest reviewers—Dr. Michele Twigg and Dr. Karen Powell Sears, Formatting—Angie Mroczka, Photographer—Sandy Aldieri (Perceptions Photography), Student graphic artists and leader—Maura, Klaudia, Amy, and Josh. And to any and all whom I may have missed who provided support to me in some way with the development of this book.

Last and not least: I want to thank everyone who completed this program and provided me feedback. Your belief in me and your commitment to the process made this book possible.

Foreword

Dear Doug,

I've been dieting most, if not all, my adult life. How tiring! I have, at times, called myself a professional dieter because it always seems as though I'm trying to find the next best diet on the market I should try. I usually get bored after reaching my goal, return to my old habits, and gain 25 pounds before I realize it's even happened. When I tell you that I've gained and lost 25 pounds at least 10 times in 20 years, I'm not kidding. Lately, I don't feel as though my body metabolizes anything.

I exercise on a regular basis. I'm a cardio girl, and eat the food suggested on whatever diet plan I'm following. I always lose weight if I keep doing cardio on a regular schedule, six to seven days a week, 45 minutes to an hour a day. I never really thought I should have to follow any type of maintenance plan because I exercise. I love to eat, I love food, I love to cook, and I love to go out. My life, as a whole, has been to diet; exercise; lose weight; exercise; go back to eating what I want; blame the holiday, work, travel, stress, et cetera, et cetera. Then I go to bed and wake up needing to lose 25 pounds. It is truly a vicious cycle. I want to learn how to lose weight, exercise, and keep it off forever. Can you help?

Patricia

Dear Patricia,

I understand your problem. You're not alone. I've heard time and time again from men and women who have had success dieting only to gain the weight back in a short period of time. Unfortunately, dieting alone is not the way to a fit, healthy, and youthful body. Your weight loss program must be comprehensive in order to be successful and lead to a healthy lifestyle, which is free of fad dieting. I recommend you try *The Perfect Scale—The Ultimate Fat Loss System.*

This 12-week program incorporates nutrition, exercise, stress management, hydration, sleep, and planning to create a synergistic approach, which will ignite your metabolism by shedding unproductive and unattractive body fat while adding attractive calorie burning, lean muscle. Any effort to change your body without including all the components I've mentioned will fall short in the long term. Follow the program, and in 12 weeks you'll have a lean, efficient, and healthy body that you'll be proud of. Keep in touch.

Doug

Doug,

OMG! I've been following *ThePerfectScale—The Ultimate Fat Loss System*, and I can't believe how terrific I feel, and must admit, look. For the first time in my life, I can actually see and feel muscles in my body that I didn't even know were there. People, mostly women, comment all the time that they love my arms, and ask me how they can get them. It feels really good to be an inspiration to others. Following the plan is challenging at times, but when you get these results, it's all worth the effort. The program really works. When people ask, I tell them you have to look at it as if it's a short-term investment for long-term results. Now I'm a solid size four, and I never thought at age 45, I would be here. I honestly spent 12 weeks accomplishing what I've been trying to do for 25 years.

Patricia

Dear Doug,

What happened to the good old days? I've been an athlete most of my life. I played sports in high school: I was honorable mention all-state in football, and the captain of my baseball team. While in college, I played intramural sports every semester. I went to work in corporate America after graduation, but still managed to stay fit. I joined an adult basketball league, my department softball team, and entered local 5Ks when I could. After getting married and having two kids, I became a bit of a weekend warrior. I coached my kids' sports teams through the years, but didn't get much exercise other than that.

My waistband has expanded, and I'm soft all over. I now know why they call it a beer belly. I've lost weight a couple of times. Once I took second in the office's biggest loser contest. Slowly, the weight came back, and it seemed like there wasn't a thing I could do about it. The kids are gone, so I get to the gym a few times a week. I do my same old routine and walk on the treadmill. I try to run, but I hurt my Achilles tendon. I'm pissed off, and I want to be healthy again. I know I can't get my 32 inch waist back, but do you think I could drop 50 pounds? Maybe try one of those mud runs? What do you think?

Bob

Dear Bob,

If you commit to this program, you'll lose at least 25 pounds of fat in three months and have the knowledge to stay fit for the rest of your life. That alone will turn back the clock, and you'll be ready to lace up your sneakers. You'll have to learn how and when to eat, but you'll never be hungry, and you'll always feel great. Since you were once an athlete and you currently go to the gym, the exercise component should be a piece of cake. Lastly, I will educate you on fat loss and how each component of fat loss plays a big part in your success. Get started right away, stay focused and consistent, and results are around the corner.

Doug

Dear Doug,

Are you kidding me? I can't believe it took me this long to do your program. I can't remember the last time I felt this great. I look pretty damn good, too! No more belly for me! I don't even need my Type 2 diabetes medicine anymore; my high blood pressure medicine dosage has been cut in half, and my doctor plans to take me off it in a few months when I go for a physical. But even better I know how to really take care of myself. I know how to eat, exercise, and I know how to eat out when I travel. Now I'm aware of how much sleep I get, and I make sure I stay hydrated and manage my stress. I know running is not part of your program, so I'm going to start slow and build so I can do a mud run race in September. Thanks again for giving me my life back.

The New Bob

Introduction

OUR WEIGHT PROBLEM

Let's face it, America; we have a weight problem, a big, fat weight problem. Two-thirds of Americans are obese or overweight. Sadly, 10% of our population is super obese. Over 20 million Americans have been diagnosed with type 2 diabetes, while another 8 million have gone undiagnosed. An estimated 80 million people, one out of three adults, are pre-diabetic, and one of three adults has prehypertension. Nearly 75 million people suffer from high blood pressure, and over a million people die each year from lifestyle diseases.[1] Meanwhile, the diet and exercise industries are bringing in record revenues. The market is flooded with weight loss drugs, surgeries, diets, exercise videos, and new fitness modalities. We've gone from CrossFit to Zumba, and we're still fat.

Let me ask you a question. If so much money is being spent on getting healthy, then why are we getting bigger and bigger? Why do most people who diet fail? Why do 90% of those who lose weight, put the weight back on? Why haven't you been successful losing weight and keeping it off? I can tell you why—your answers to weight loss are incomplete.

---

1   "The vast majority of American adults are overweight or obese, and weight is a growing problem among US children." Institute for Health Metrics and Evaluation. Accessed December 2017. http://www.healthdata.org/news-release/vast-majority-american-adults-are-overweight-or-obese-and-weight-growing-problem-among; National Center for Chronic Disease Prevention and Health Promotion. "Estimates of Diabetes and Its Burden in the United States." National Diabetes Statistics Report, 2017. Accessed December 2017. http://www.diabetes.org/assets/pdfs/basics/cdc-statistics-report-2017.pdf; "Division for Heart Disease and Stroke Prevention." Centers for Disease Control and Prevention. June 16, 2016. Accessed December 2017. https://www.cdc.gov/dhdsp/data_statistics/fact_sheets/fs_bloodpressure.htm; "High Blood Pressure." Centers for Disease Control and Prevention. November 13, 2017. Accessed December 2017. https://www.cdc.gov/bloodpressure/index.htm.

Most people pursue weight loss from one or two avenues: nutrition and exercise. However, people don't pursue *good* nutrition; instead they follow some ridiculous diet, often low in calories. With exercise, people most often engage in some sort of cardiovascular activity. While cardiovascular activity such as walking, running, and elliptical are exercise, those types of exercise rank at the bottom of the totem pole for weight loss. These two avenues, nutrition and exercise, aren't bad, but people are implementing them incorrectly. This often leads to frustration, which eventually leads to failure. A successful weight loss program includes much more than these tandem actions. A successful approach to weight loss should not only include nutrition and exercise, but hydration, sleep, stress management, and planning. Yes, planning. Before I get into all of that, let me tell you a little bit about me.

MY SYSTEM AND EXPERTISE

My name is Doug Dorsey, known as the Fitness Professor. I'm 50 years old, a fat loss coach, a healthy lifestyle transformation expert, community college professor, and father of two. Health and fitness has been a lifetime interest of mine. As a personal trainer and fitness coach for the past 10 years, I've helped people shed fat, lose weight, add muscle, and obtain any fitness goal they desired. I formally began in the industry by training natural female figure and body building competitors—those freakishly lean bodies you've seen wearing a bathing suit parading around the stage. Several of my clients made it to the professional level. But for the most part, I have helped hundreds of everyday people lose weight and live incredible lives.

In my studios, we help people work towards achieving their weight and fat loss goals, and we love it. Over the years, I've read all the available books and studied the research; I've tested the theories and philosophies on my own body and with clients. I've seen failures, and I've seen successes. I've lost weight, gained weight, added muscle, and have run a couple half-marathons myself. Through my exhaustive efforts to extend my knowledge in this area and my hands-on experience, I've learned what works and what doesn't. With this knowledge, I've created *ThePerfectScale—The Ultimate Fat*

Loss System. Using this system, I've educated people on how to be successful in the fat loss arena. Clients from all walks of life have been successful in implementing *ThePerfectScale—The Ultimate Fat Loss System*. I've applied this knowledge and developed a fool-proof, how-to guide to help you be successful as well.

While you may have tried other methodologies, you haven't had an opportunity to follow a comprehensive weight loss/lifestyle program like this previously because this is the first of its kind. With *ThePerfectScale—The Ultimate Fat Loss System*, you'll learn the key components to improving your metabolism and how to manage each component so your body will be burning fat 24 hours a day. I introduce you to a new scale that will track your progress daily, and allow you to throw your old scale in the basement. The programs you heard of or tried have been incomplete. No wonder only 10% of the people who try to lose weight are successful. Through trial and error, stubbornness and luck, the 10% that were successful figured it out. Well, I've taken out the guess work and the misinformation, as I clear up all the clutter and misinformation in the media. This is the last weight loss effort you will ever need to make. The proof is in the pudding. Everyone that has completed this program has lost a significant amount of body fat. By significant, I mean on average between 25 to 33 percent of their body fat, while adding muscle. That's life changing. Look at some of the client results on my website, www.TheFitnessProfessor.com Most of my clients aren't interested in shedding their anonymity by displaying their photos to the world, and I respect that, so some of their faces and pictures will be missing. This program isn't about vanity: it's about losing fat and keeping it off. However, major visual changes are one of the benefits.

Now it simply becomes your turn to act. I guarantee that if you follow *ThePerfectScale—The Ultimate Fat Loss System*, you will turn the clock back 10 years. You will lose weight, you will feel and look better, and you will reduce or eliminate the medications that you're on. You will understand how to live a healthy lifestyle, and you will never need to diet again. Most importantly, you will learn how to take care of your body. This is my promise to you, and if you are not successful, I will give you your money back. Go to ThePerfectScale.

com to see my money-back guarantee offer. You only have one life to live, and you're entitled to do it any way you want. If you want to live a healthier life and educate yourself, then you've purchased the right book. Don't hesitate, or try some other program, because there's none better.

WHAT YOU NEED TO COMMIT TO BEFORE YOU START

Regardless of your goal, whether you want to lose 20 or 200 pounds, get off meds, feel better, look better, or simply live a healthy lifestyle, *ThePerfectScale—The Ultimate Fat Loss System* is the one and only program you'll ever need. In order to get started, you'll have to put aside your past beliefs about weight loss, exercise, and nutrition. Not that they all may be wrong, although some things you've been reading and doing are wrong, but in order to follow the program properly, you need to let go of all of your preconceived ideas about weight loss. I know, I know. You heard it on *The Dr. Oz Show*, and Jillian Michaels says, and in the last issue of *Muscle and Fitness*, and my trainer, who helped me lose 25 pounds, says ... yada, yada, yada.

I get it. It's hard to put aside things that you have heard, and maybe that even have helped you be successful in the past. Honestly, I've learned a lot from those sources myself. I've watched *The Dr. Oz Show* and read his books, and Jillian is a leader and an icon in this industry. I would have never done yoga if it weren't for her DVD's. I've incorporated some of the same beliefs and principles in *ThePerfectScale—The Ultimate Fat Loss System*. But in order to be successful, you must follow this system completely. It's that simple. You can't be half-hearted in your approach or semi-commit to it, nor do 50% of this system, together with 30% of the Paleo diet, plus 20% Insanity workout, or some other combination. I know some of you will, and that's your prerogative. The reality is you're free to do so. The other reality is you purchased this book, which a system. A system which people have tremendous success when following and only so-so results by self-altering with their personal "knowledge." Don't alter or reinvent the wheel. The work has been done for you. All you have to do is follow it as designed.

Along with putting aside your past beliefs, you must understand that fat is the enemy. In our society, it's easy to talk about weight and weight loss, but several things make up your weight and most weight loss. Weight is easy to measure. Step on a scale and a number appears, plot that number on a chart and you fall into one of three categories: you're either fit, overweight, or obese. Chances are even if you're at normal weight; you may have too much body fat.

The truth of the matter is fat kills. It wreaks havoc on your body, your organs, and lifestyle. It's also unattractive and depressing. Fat is the enemy, and *ThePerfectScale—The Ultimate Fat Loss System* puts a bulls eye on it; it's relentless in its pursuit to minimize it. Before I explain how we do it, you should have an understanding of where fat comes from and its purpose. Fat is stored energy. Fat serves several vital functions to the body. It builds healthy cells, helps the body use vitamins, forms a protective cushion for organs, and also provides energy. We need body fat, and if it gets too low, we run into health problems.

Excess fat is an abundance of stored energy that you (yes, you!) accumulated by taking in more food, which is energy, than you burned, which is movement. It's that simple. You ate more than you needed, so your body stored it. Your body thinks there will be a need for it later. Otherwise, why would you have eaten it? Your body doesn't know it tastes good, it's mom's cooking, junk food, or super-sized. Your body just knows energy. You gave your body energy, which is food, but your body didn't need it, because you didn't move enough.

The only ways to eliminate the stored energy, or fat, without getting it sucked out surgically, is to consume less energy than you need or to move more. That is a very simple explanation of how fat accumulates in the body. Is it more complicated than that? Could be. Does it have to be? No. Just note, too much fat is bad, and when you've accumulated it, you must get rid of it. Don't look to lose weight; lose fat. (From now on, when you see the words weight loss it means fat loss). So, how do we lose fat? We improve your metabolism. Your metabolism is your fat burning clock.

This system, remember it's a **system**, will improve your metabolism. At a network marketing meeting I once attended, I heard a speaker say, "Some will; some won't; so what; who's next?" I thought it sounded rather cold at the time, but at this stage in my life, I understand. I want to help those who "will." If you're one of those people—let's get going! If you're not, I wish you the best on your journey. When you're ready, so am I. I'm always ready to assist people on this journey. All you have to do is follow the program, and you will see proven results. My website provides you with a myriad of free and some fee-based support, so you can be successful implementing *ThePerfectScale—The Ultimate Fat Loss System*. Go to my website www.TheFitnessProfessor.com and download the free guide that accompanies this book. As you read along, you will use it to create your custom program.

Chapter 1 — What Is a System?

A system is a set of principles or procedures according to which something is done, designed to be automatic and operate consistently every time it's put into operation.

Think back to when you were an infant. Do you remember the first time you ate? Of course not. How about your first bowel movement? Don't remember that either? As a newborn, you had no idea that the food, breast milk or formula, you were consuming was going to nourish your body and pass the waste out of the other end. Did you will that to happen? No. Once you consumed the food, your digestive system took over. Your digestive system is responsible for taking food and turning it into energy and nutrients that allow the body to function, grow, and repair itself. Without giving you a complicated biology lesson, briefly, here's how your digestive system works.

1. You ingest food or liquids through your mouth. Then you chew it, swallow it, and pass it into your esophagus, which carries it from your mouth to your stomach.

2. The stomach mixes the food with digestive juices, and slowly empties its contents into the small intestine.

3. To help with further digestion, the small intestine mixes the food with more digestive juices; this time from the pancreas, liver, and intestine. The walls of the small intestine allow the digested nutrients to be absorbed into the bloodstream. Then the blood delivers the nutrients to the rest of the body.

4. The waste products of the digestive process are pushed into the large intestine, which then absorbs any of the remaining nutrients and changes the waste from liquid to stool. The rectum then pushes the stool out of the body.

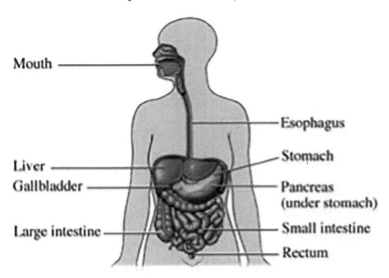

Mouth

Esophagus

Stomach

Liver

Gallbladder

Pancreas
(under stomach)

Large intestine

Small intestine

Rectum

Figure 1. Digestive System Parts (Source: "Digestive system diagram." Money. Accessed December 2017. http://civicmediaproject.org/works/money/digestive-system-diagram.)

It's incredible to think that all of this happened automatically, and all you did was simply consume food. Your digestive system is amazing. You know what else is amazing? Your body. It has many major systems that operate automatically to keep you alive and well:

1. Cardiovascular System
2. Circulatory System
3. Digestive System
4. Endocrine System
5. Immune System
6. Lymphatic System
7. Muscular Systems
8. Nervous System
9. Reproductive System
10. Respiratory System
11. Skeletal System
12. Urinary System

Again, these systems operate automatically and work together to keep you alive. Think about your car, it operates based on the interworking of a variety of systems. It has an electrical, emissions, exhaust, fuel, transmission, and brake system to name a few. We simply open the door, put the key in the ignition, turn the switch, and drive away. These systems, however, must work together to allow your car to operate properly so you can get to your destination without breaking down. The best thing about systems is they are automatic. Because of these systems, you can eliminate making a ton of decisions.

When we eat food, we don't have to decide where it should go next. The process takes care of itself. When we step on the brake pedal, it applies pressure to the breaks and the car slows down. We don't have to think about it unless, of course, it is broken.

When any of our systems don't work, an analysis is done, the faulty component is found, it is repaired or replaced, and the system is off and running again.

The Perfect Scale—The Ultimate Fat Loss System is similar to these other systems in that it has several key components and it works automatically to burn fat. A diagram of *The Perfect Scale—The Ultimate Fat Loss System* looks like this.

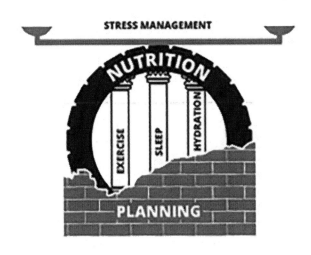

I will spend a chapter explaining each component in detail, as well as its role in the fat loss system, but for now I will briefly describe each one:

PLANNING

Planning is the foundation of the fat loss system. If you do not plan what you're going to eat, when you're going to exercise, and how you're going to manage your stress, your fat loss efforts are doomed! Imagine building a house without a foundation; it's destined to fail, so is your fat loss effort without planning.

NUTRITION

Nutrition is the wheel. For the fat loss system to work, the wheel of nutrition must be in motion. Your fat loss isn't going anywhere without this wheel to propel it forward.

EXERCISE

Exercise or movement is one of three spokes in the wheel. It supports the wheel of nutrition by burning fat and adding muscle. Exercise is the sizzle on the steak, or the accelerant to your fat loss. It speeds up the wheel of nutrition with fat loss. By itself, it has a minimal impact on fat loss.

HYDRATION

Hydration is the second spoke in the wheel. It is a vital part of your daily nutrition and will allow you to function and exercise at peak capacity. It also helps your body and organs function properly so you can burn maximum fat.

SLEEP

Sleep is the third spoke in the wheel. Proper sleep allows the body to heal and regenerate so it's able to perform and move (exercise) with limited fatigue. Sleep also allows for proper nutrition by limiting the cravings and desires to eat fat gaining foods

STRESS MANAGEMENT

Since it is imperative that you manage your stress in order to lose fat, stress management is at the top of the diagram. Stress will disrupt the entire fat loss process if left unchecked. If stress is out of line, it will put a weight on either end of the stress bar and send the wheel of nutrition rolling off its foundation.

ThePerfectScale—The Ultimate Fat Loss System integrates all the components required to increase your metabolism and burn fat. The best part is it's automatic. The system runs your fat loss for you. You simply run the system!

Chapter 2—America's Weight Loss

Now that you know what the fat loss system looks like, or at least what the components are, let's talk about America's fat loss system.

Let's say you had a problem, any type of problem, with your car, home, health, or an appliance and part of the solution included spending $300 toward solving the problem. What would you do if 20 years later the problem still exists or is in fact, worse? How about if the problem has multiplied threefold, and now you're spending $600 instead of $300 toward finding a solution? Would you stop wasting your money? Would you look for an alternative solution? Would you think that you were scammed or sold snake oil? Well, that's exactly what's happening in the weight loss industry.

According to the U.S. Food and Drug Administration, Americans spent an estimated $30 billion in 1992 on all types of diet programs and products, including diet foods and drinks. According to Market Data Enterprises, the marketing research firm tracking diet products and programs, Americans spent more than $60 billion in 2012 trying to lose weight. Do the math. In 20 years, we've basically doubled the money we're spending on weight loss, and the problem tripled during the same time!!! Sounds insane, doesn't it?

According to figure 2, in 1990, no state had more than 15 percent obesity rates. In fact, 10 states had an obesity rate of less than 10 percent. By 2000, that was history. There were zero states with an obesity rate under 10 percent, and 23 states had a prevalence of obesity between 20 and 24 percent. By the turn of the century, no state had an obesity rate equal to or greater than 25 percent.

By 2010, no state had a prevalence of obesity *less* than 20 percent! Thirty-six states, or two-thirds of the country, had a prevalence equal to or greater than 25 percent and 12 states had a prevalence of obesity equal to or greater than 30 percent. We're growing at an alarming rate. Using these same numbers and projecting forward, by 2020, nearly every state will have a prevalence of obesity greater than 25 percent and half of the country will be over 30 percent! The scary part about these numbers is we're talking about obesity. If the maps included overweight people, we'd be talking about two-thirds to three-quarters of our population. The more we spend on weight loss, the fatter we seem to become. Would you agree that this is insane?

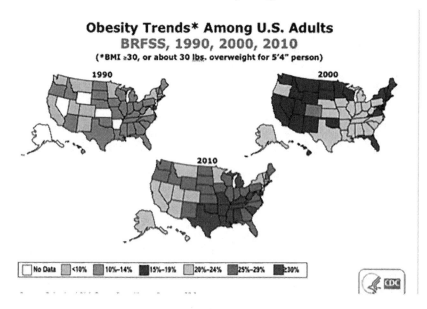

Figure 2. Obesity Trends from CDC (Source: Behavioral Risk Factor Surveillance System, US Centers for Disease Control and Prevention.)

What we're doing isn't working. Maybe we should just stop spending money, and the problem will go away, but I doubt it. Overweight and obesity conditions are the second leading cause of preventable death in the United States. Based on the current trends, it will overtake smoking as the leading cause of preventable deaths in a short period of time! That statement is worth repeating: Based on the current trends, overweight and obesity conditions will overtake smoking as the leading cause of preventable deaths in a short period of time! The leading cause of preventable deaths will soon be FAT!!!

So how did we get so fat, and why aren't current weight loss efforts working? Let's address these issues one at a time.

So how did we get so fat, and why do we keep growing fatter? In order for such an epidemic to occur, there has to be multiple causes, meaning it is a combination of these causes that set us on this catastrophic, deadly path. These causes are not in any particular order.

#1 INCREASED CALORIC INTAKE

Between portion distortion, eating out, and our increased consumption of food, we are simply eating too much. The average daily caloric intake per capita in the United States is 3,700 calories per person. Economic research data from the United States Department of Agriculture suggests that average daily caloric intake has increased by 24.5 percent or about 530 calories between 1970 and 2000. Let's do the math. 530 calories x 7 days = 3,710 calories per week. 3,500 calories = 1 pound. We are consuming 1 pound of additional food per week compared to 1970!

#2 WE'RE EATING OUT MORE OFTEN

This will be addressed later in the book. However, in March of 2015, spending on dining out overtook grocery store purchases for the first time ever! The average American adult buys a meal or snack from a restaurant almost six times a week. Eating out leads to the consumption of too many calories, often from increased sugar, fat, and carbohydrate consumption. Fast food is cheap, and this cheap food often comes in large quantities. While the caloric count is high and it's loaded with fat, sugar and salt, often the quality of the food isn't very good.

#3 WE'RE CONSUMING TOO MUCH SUGAR

When the country went to a low-fat diet, we replaced fat with sugar. According to the American Heart Association, women should not consume more than 6 teaspoons (100 calories) and men should not consume more than 9 teaspoons (150 calories) of sugar per day. However, more than 70 percent of Americans eat at least 22 teaspoons of added sugar daily according to the Harvard School of Public Health. This increased sugar appears on our waist line.

#4 INCREASED CONSUMPTION OF PROCESSED FOODS

We have foods today that didn't even exist 20 years ago. Many of these processed, convenient foods offer little or no nutrition and are loaded with salt, fat, and sugar.

#5 WE'RE SLEEPING LESS

Americans average six and a half hours of sleep at night compared to the nearly eight hour 1942 average. Medical studies have related a lack of sleep to health problems and cognitive impairment. Therefore, experts typically recommend seven to nine hours of sleep for adults. This lack of sleep has had a direct effect on how we eat.

#6 WE'VE BECOME A CONVENIENCE CULTURE

This means inferior quality nutrition, increased caloric intake, and less movement.

#7 INCREASED MEDICATIONS

Some prescription drugs cause weight gain. Almost half of Americans take at least one prescription drug. Ten percent use five or more! Of the two-thirds of people in the United States who are overweight, many take drugs to treat obesity-linked conditions such as diabetes, high blood pressure, and depression, but many of those medicines cause weight gain. There's an oxymoron for you: "I'm overweight which is causing health problems, so I'm going to take a drug that's going to continue to cause me to gain weight but hide the health problem." Weight loss isn't the only thing we do wrong in this country.

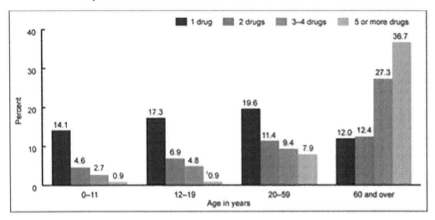

Figure 3. Percentage of prescription drugs use in the past month (Source: CDC/ NCHS, National Health and Nutrition Examination Survey.)

#8 STRESS

A sizable number of Americans say stress causes some unhealthy behaviors like lying awake at night rather than sleeping (Forty-two percent admit stress has led to lack of sleep) and overeating unhealthy foods (Thirty-three percent admit doing this because of stress).[1]

#9 WE SIT TOO MUCH

Either in a car on the way to work, in a chair while at work, or on the sofa watching TV or surfing the internet, this lack of movement causes us to burn fewer and fewer calories. The average American watches five hours of television a day! While this may be great for Netflix, it's horrible for your waistline. We don't even go out to shop for clothes or groceries anymore. We sit, click buttons, and they appear at the door!

There are other reasons why we're fat, but I think you get the idea.

---

1   "Stress in America Report." American Psychological Association. Accessed December 2017. http://www.apa.org/news/press/releases/stress/index.aspx.

Let's now address the problem of weight loss efforts not working. I define working as success. I define success as losing weight and keeping it off, at least most of it. Would you consider a marriage successful if it ended in divorce? No, you wouldn't. Then so too, if you lose weight, but gain the weight back, you wouldn't consider it a success. When it comes to losing weight and keeping it off, the success rate is 10 percent.

A 10 percent success rate is dismal. In any grading system, that's an F minus. Sixty-five billion dollars spent, and we have an F minus rating! Something is wrong. So why don't our weight loss efforts work? First, let's take a look at the typical weight loss scenario.

Bob or Mary has thought about losing weight. They will either try whatever diet their friend, neighbor, or co-worker is doing or has done that appears successful. Whether the diet is right for them doesn't matter. If that friend, neighbor, or co-worker is doing a workout program to lose weight, then Bob or Mary will join the bandwagon also. So they may start walking, join a Zumba class, go to the gym, or purchase P90X. If Bob or Mary does not start doing what their friend, neighbor, or co-worker is doing, they will find a diet program they heard about or their doctor recommended. They may even do some research on a particular diet.

Unfortunately, once they begin the research process, here's where the failure begins. Let's take a look at some of these diet programs that we've seen over the years. We've got the Atkins Diet, the Zone Diet, Vegetarian Diet, Vegan Diet, Weight Watchers Diet, South Beach Diet, Raw Food Diet, and the Mediterranean Diet. Not done yet. There's also the Grapefruit Diet, the Skinny Bitch Diet, the Three Hour Diet, the Best Life Diet, the Blood Type Diet, the Fat Flush Diet, the Caveman Diet, French Women Don't Get Fat Diet, the Glycemic Index Diet, Macrobiotic Diet, the Hormone Diet, New Beverly Hills Diet, and the Master's Cleanse Diet.

Still not done. How about the HCG Diet, the Vision Diet, the Eight Hour Diet, the Dessert with Breakfast Diet, the Cookie Diet, the Baby Food Diet. Still more. We've got the Belly Fat Cure Diet, Cheater's Diet, and the Carbs Lover Diet. Don't forget we also have

Weight Watchers, Nutri-System, Jenny Craig, LA Weight Loss, and on, and on and on.

How in the world are they supposed to choose a diet with all these options? Somehow, they do.

At this point in our hypothetical, Bob and Mary start spending five hours at the gym or pounding the pavement, and they begin their chosen program. However, the diet program is too low in calories, which results not only in losing weight, but also muscle. This is the first step of long-term failure and the beginning of being caught in the weight loss/weight gain, pick-a-new-diet roller coaster. But before they get caught in the cycle, they lose five, 10, or even 20 pounds. Congratulations, Bob and Mary! They begin fitting into things they haven't worn in a while and people are starting to notice. They might make it to month number two with similar or continued positive results.

At some point though, "it" kicks in. They start missing things. They want pizza, bread, cookies, pasta, soda, etc. Because of the low-calorie diet, they're hungry, and their diet food doesn't taste good any longer. No longer able to resist the temptations, they indulge in unhealthy food, but only in moderation. However, moderation eventually leads to indulgence. The extended time doing cardio continues, until life gets in the way. Eventually, the weight is back on.

They're now a little depressed. Also, their ego just took a hit because they failed. Maybe this is the second or third time that they failed to lose weight. Unfortunately, they don't even realize that they've lost muscle—calorie-burning, youthful-looking muscle—the fountain of youth they just lost on their diet, causing them to be less prepared to handle the junk food they are now consuming. Guess what happens? They start to gain more weight, more fat, to be exact. They go to the doctor for their six month or annual check-up, and the doctor says, "Bob/Mary, what's going on? You've got to lose some weight." They walk out the door, and their mind starts to go through the diet list all over again, and the process repeats itself.

Basically, diets are an incomplete way to lose weight and keep it off. If you're going to keep the weight off, you need a comprehensive approach. After the diet, you regain weight because the diet is not sustainable. Even if you are successful on a diet plan, most plans don't show you how to maintain your weight loss while you're in weight maintenance. People often go back to their unhealthy habits and the weight usually returns, at least 90 percent of the time.

Additionally, most people are using the wrong tools to help them lose weight. Most people still rely on the scale. The scale is one of the worst tools for fat loss. I repeat, the scale is one of the worst tools EVER for fat loss. Take it and throw it down the basement stairs. Bring it out only after you've reached your fat loss goals.

Why is the scale a horrible fat loss tool?

Number one, it measures weight not fat. Remember fat is the enemy, muscle is your friend. The typical scale cannot tell you how much fat you're losing; however, some of the new scales do. I do, however, question their accuracy.

Number two, the scale is more of a de-motivator than a motivator. You eat well all day or week; you've exercised a few times, not enough, but more than usual; you get on the scale and you haven't lost a pound or maybe you've lost just one. It's not what you expected, and you're discouraged. Time to eat. Your plan goes out the window.

Number three, the scale does not measure the components of fat loss. You need to track how you're doing in the areas that lead to fat loss. That is the most important thing to measure. The fat loss will come if you do the right things. So, do the right things and forget the scale. I will introduce you to an easy tracking system that beats a scale any day, and it's free.

In terms of wrong tools, you shouldn't trust food trackers. They are yet another waste of time. While they've come a long way and are much improved, they still aren't 100 percent accurate, and it's difficult to make the food you consume fit into the programs. For example, try entering your homemade turkey chili into a food tracker. Another problem is they are used post-eating. People eat all day, then try hard to remember what they ate, and then have to plug it into a program to see what their calorie count is for the day. That's backwards. You wouldn't take your paycheck, spend your money, and then try to figure out if you spent too much at the end of the week or month. To manage your money properly, you would create a budget initially, and then follow the budget.

Additionally, food trackers are time consuming. If your goal is fat loss, you should know what foods to consume and what quantities are appropriate. No need to waste time tracking it. The time should be spent on planning your food and preparing it.

Lastly, exercise gadgets don't help either. Fitbits and the other calorie tracking devices are simply unnecessary for fat loss. Yes, it's great to exercise, and it should be the part of any fat loss program; however, the tracking devices are often inaccurate. If you're counting steps, you're measuring the wrong thing. Walking is one of the least effective forms of exercise for fat loss. If you're exercising for fat loss properly, the benefit comes after the exercise is over. That's what you want to measure, but it's virtually impossible without going to a lab. These devices are also expensive, and the money could be used on fitness equipment and weights for your home. Spend your money purchasing fitness DVDs or learning how to exercise properly so you don't need to track your calories. Very seldom do you see a fit person with one of these devices on their wrist. Until there is one designed to support *ThePerfectScale—The Ultimate Fat Loss System*, stay away from them. Stay tuned, it's coming soon!

So, avoid spending time or money on these gadgets or diets. They've proven themselves incapable of handling the weight loss problem in America. Do you need any more proof than $60,000,000,000 for a 10 percent success rate?

Chapter 3—Why Fat Loss and Not Weight Loss?

You now know that billions of dollars are spent on various weight loss methods that simply don't work. Yes, some people have had success. However, with a 10 percent success rate, I'd say they were lucky because they managed to hang in there long enough to realize how to find success in the weight loss arena. In order to track success, The National Weight Control Registry (NWCR) investigates the characteristics of individuals who have succeeded at long-term weight loss. They are currently tracking over 10,000 individuals who have lost a significant amount of weight and kept it off for long periods of time. This registry can serve as an example of successful weight loss. Some of the same findings identified by the registry are incorporated in *ThePerfectScale—The Ultimate Fat Loss System.*

Those who have been successful modified their food intake, in some way, to lose weight. They increased their physical activity. They exercised on a consistent basis. They ate breakfast every day. They watched minimal amounts of television, and they weighed themselves at least once a week. Like many organizations, the studies the NWCR focuses on pertain to weight. While I understand weight is a problem (and it's much easier to record, document, and track), weight, ultimately, is not the problem—fat is. Your weight consists of fat free mass or muscle, and fat mass, which we refer to as fat. Fat causes metabolic syndrome, obesity, disease, and premature deaths. Muscle has nothing to do with it. I repeat. Muscle has nothing to do with it. In fact, muscle helps to ward off both obesity and disease. It also contributes to your quality of life. The problem with most diets and weight loss efforts is that you lose precious muscle along with some fat, so your body is less efficient when you stop dieting than when you started. This contributes significantly to eventual weight gain.

The first thing you must understand is fat is the enemy, not your weight. In our society, it's easy to talk about weight and weight loss. As stated previously, weight is easy to measure. You get on a scale, and a number appears. Plot that number on a chart, and bingo, you're fit, overweight, or obese. Chances are, if you're overweight or obese, you have too much body fat. That's what caused the problem to start with. Your goal should be to lose only fat, but instead you focus on losing weight. You get back on the scale, the scale goes down, and you feel successful. Chances are, you lost a little fat, and plenty of muscle. When you stop dieting, the scale goes right back up. That's one of the worst things you could have done to your body. Why? You'll find out shortly. Let's stick to the fat. The truth of the matter is excess fat kills. It wreaks havoc on your body, organs, and lifestyle, not to mention it's unattractive and depressing. *ThePerfectScale* puts a bull's-eye on fat, and it's relentless in its pursuit to reduce it.

Before I explain how we do it, you should have an understanding of the purpose of fat in your body. Fat is one of the three required macronutrients humans need to live. The other two are protein and carbohydrates. We must consume fat every day, or we will develop serious health problems. Fat serves several functions in the body.

- Fat absorbs and stores certain vitamins. Without fat, the absorption of Vitamins A, D, E, and K are restricted, and eventually a breakdown will occur. These vitamins are vital to our vision, bones, and cellular health.

- Fat is a secondary source of energy. Our primary energy source is carbohydrates; thus, when carbohydrates aren't present in our system, or have been used up, the body turns to fat for additional energy.

- Fat helps to maintain body temperature by insulating the body and maintaining its core temperature.

- Fat helps to protect the body as the stored fat surrounds vital organs. If, for some reason, you experience a sudden impact, or even severe trauma, fat will absorb as much of the shock as possible to protect vital organs, including the brain and the heart.

- Fat supports reproduction. Sex hormones are fat soluble. If a woman's body fat is too low, she'll produce less estrogen, which may lead to an abnormal menstrual cycle.

While we need fat, too much is detrimental to your health. See figure 4 for body fat ranges and recommendations. Your goal should lie somewhere in the fitness category.

ACE Body Fat % Chart		
Description	Women	Men
Essential fat	10-13%	2-5%
Athletes	14–20%	6-13%
Fitness	21–24%	14–17%
Average	25–31%	18–24%
Obese	32%+	25%+

Figure 4. Body Fat Recommendations/Guidelines (Source: "Research and Studies." ACE | Certified Personal Trainer | ACE Personal Trainer. Accessed December 2017. https://www.acefitness.org/.)

This chart shows the percentage of body fat that is acceptable in each category (the recommendations do vary by age). Ideally, you should fall in the fitness category. But regardless, this chart shows that fat is essential to your body. However while we need fat, there are good fats and bad fats. We'll discuss this in a later chapter. The good fats keep our bodies healthy and protect our hearts. The bad fats can damage our heart and increase the risk of disease. Excess body fat does the same, which is a major problem. Even if you start to consume good fats, you still can have excess fat on your body that can cause heart problems. How did you accumulate excess fat on your body? By consuming too many calories. When you consume too many calories, your body stores that food as energy to be used later.

I've stated this earlier, but I'll repeat it again because it's so important: excess fat is simply an abundance of stored energy that is accumulated by taking in more food or energy than is burned or used by movement. If you eat more than is needed, the body will store it. Since your body just knows energy, it thinks there will be a need for it later. But because you didn't move enough, you gave your body energy which it didn't need. The only way to eliminate that stored energy, without getting it removed surgically, is to move more.

I just gave a very simple example of how fat accumulates in the body. Is it more complicated than that? Could be. Does it have to be? No. Just know, excess fat is bad; you accumulated it, so you must get rid of it. Don't look to lose weight, lose fat. We'll talk about how you do that in the next chapter.

Let's take a few minutes and talk about muscle, and why it's important to your body.

- Musculoskeletal system allows for the movement of the body. Muscles work by contracting and relaxing to create movement in the action of the body, such as raising or lowering a limb. Bending a joint is possible because of skeletal muscle.

- Muscle allows us to maintain our posture and our body position. A simple view of someone with poor posture or poor body positioning identifies a lack of muscle.

- Muscle allows for the movement of fluids inside the body. This is done by smooth muscle (the gastrointestinal tract is one example of a smooth muscle), which controls the flow of fluids through an organ. These muscles are controlled unconsciously by the brain.

Muscle plays a key role in determining the number of calories you need to maintain your body at rest, known as your Basal Metabolic Rate or BMR. If you have a higher percentage of muscle compared to fat, you will require more calories. This makes muscle a natural line of defense against fat accumulation, which ultimately means it helps ward off obesity, diabetes, and metabolic syndrome. Our energy/caloric needs decrease as we lose muscle mass, so if your weight loss program causes you to lose muscle, when you get off the program, you cannot eat the same amount of food as you used to, or you'll gain weight. This is the primary reason why most weight loss efforts fail in the long run and what makes *ThePerfectScale—The Ultimate Fat Loss System* the best program available.

Not only do we focus on burning fat, but we focus on increasing muscle mass as well. This combination not only results in a more efficient body, it also makes it easier to maintain your weight once you're in a maintenance mode. It never requires you to diet or lose fat again.

Now that you understand that fat is the problem, not weight, and you know that muscle is important to your metabolic rate and keeping fat off, you're ready for an education on true fat loss.

Chapter 4—How Do You Lose Fat?

Remember, we don't want to lose weight; we want to lose fat. We never, ever, ever want to lose muscle! How do you lose fat? That's the million dollar question, or should I say, $60 billion dollar question. Let's keep it simple. I'll explain each area in detail throughout the remainder of the book.

The first way we lose fat is through eating or observing good nutrition. As I mentioned earlier, you gain fat by eating too much. The way to lose fat through food is by eating less than you need. (Note: you should never consume less than your BMR, but just less than what you need when you take your activity into account. I will explain how you figure this out in a moment.) When you consume less food than you need, your body has to resort to an alternative source for fuel. As long as you don't reduce your food consumption too low, your body will turn to fat, stored food/energy, for fuel. When it uses stored fat for fuel, your fat cells shrink, resulting in a smaller, healthier you.

How much food should you consume? You are going to need to brush up on your math skills and plug your information into the formula below to determine your Basal Metabolic Rate (BMR). You can complete this step by step in your guide.

Use the Harris–Benedict equation revised by Mifflin and St Jeor in 1990:

MEN

10 x Body weight in kilograms + 6.25 x height in centimeters - 5 x times your age in years + 5.

WOMEN

10 x Body weight in kilograms + 6.25 x height in centimeters - 5 x times your age in years - 161.

Example:

200 pound, 5 foot 10 inch, 50 year old male, moderate exerciser. BMR will be calculated as follows:

10 x (200 x.45359237) + 6.25 x (70 x 2.54) - 5 x 50 + 5

10 x 90.718474 + (6.25 x 177.8) - 250 + 5

907.18 + 1111.25 -245 = 1,773 calories

You don't have to remember high school algebra to lose fat. Just follow the step by step process in your guide.

There are some assumptions built into this formula; however, it is considered the standard when calculating BMR. If you have access to a professional with the proper equipment, they can test you to determine your BMR. Their number would be more accurate because it takes into consideration everything that's going on in your body, along with your body composition. However, the professional number won't vary significantly from the calculation you arrived at using this formula.

Your BMR is the number of calories your body requires to support vital body functions if you were only sitting on a couch for the entire day. You should never consume less than your BMR. If you're extremely overweight or obese, you should not exceed 2000-2500 calories. Your BMR is the largest number of your total energy burned each day. Remember, that's based on you sitting still all day. That number needs to be adjusted to account for energy burned sleeping, yes, even sleeping, working, exercising, and digesting food.

To get your Total Daily Energy Expenditure or TDEE, take your BMR, 1,773, and multiply it by your activity multiplier as noted in figure 5.

Activity Multipliers	
1.2	Sedentary; little or no exercise
1.375	Lightly Active; light exercise 1-3 days per week
1.55	Moderately Active; moderate exercise 3-5 days per week
1.725	Very Active; hard exercise 6-7 days per week
1.9	Extremely Active; hard daily exercise

Figure 5. Activity Multipliers (Source: "CALORIES (kilocalories or kcals)." Ecoculture Village's Health Happiness Longevity. Accessed December 2017. http://www.ecoculturevillage.org/healthhappinesslongevity/calories-kilocalories-or-kcals/.)

I am a moderate exerciser, five days a week, so I use 1.55.

I need 1,773 calories daily, so I multiply that by 1.55 and get 2,748. If I'm trying to lose weight, I will consume 2,048 to 2,248 calories daily to create a caloric deficit, meaning I'm not taking in as many calories as I need. My body will utilize stored fat for the remainder of the energy needed, hence, fat loss. That is how you loss fat with food.

Another way to lose fat is to exercise. Contrary to popular belief, exercise alone does not cause much fat loss. However, it does play a role in fat loss when combined with proper nutrition. Since exercisers often cancel out the calories they burned by eating more, a phenomenon called Compensation Theory, exercise alone does not result in fat loss.

Although I have trained for and have run two half-marathons, I am not a runner. I was running up to 15-20 miles a week during training for each race. The races were nine years apart, and each time, I gained weight during training. I totally subscribed to the Compensation Theory. Keep in mind, exercise is calories out and that counts for something. Exercising for fat loss increases what we call EPOC, Excess Post-Exercise Oxygen Consumption. EPOC is the increased rate of oxygen intake after exercise that is needed to erase the body's oxygen deficit, caused by exercising strenuously.

The increased oxygen is used to restore the body to a resting state, called homeostasis. During the period of EPOC, which can last up to 36 hours, depending on the intensity of the exercise, your body's metabolism will continue to burn more calories than when at complete rest. The calorie burn helps contribute to the calorie deficit needed to burn fat.

So there you have it.

That's how you burn fat: by employing nutrition and exercise or as I like to call it Nexercise™. The two go hand in hand.

Most people know that this is the best way to lose weight. However, they generally approach each the wrong way. We'll clear this up in their perspective chapters. While Nexercise™ is important, we're not done yet. We can burn fat other ways.

A third way to burn fat is during sleep. It's true that your body burns calories while you're sleeping. Your body burns calories by sustaining vital functions of the body, repairing cells, pumping blood, and maintain your temperature all while you're resting. You're probably thinking what difference does it make if I'm sleeping or sitting on the couch, my body will still burn calories. That's true. The difference is in how you behave when you have had a proper amount of sleep, seven to nine hours, and how you behave when you haven't. This will be discussed in further detail in chapter 10.

A recent study from the University of Chicago compared the weight loss results of people sleeping eight and a half hours per night verses those only sleeping five and a half hours per night. In both groups, participants consumed the same number of calories per day, about 1,450. While both groups lost about six and a half pounds, more than half of that weight was fat for the well-rested people compared to only one-fourth for those getting the reduced number of hours of sleep. That means that three-fourths of their weight loss was muscle, which is a definite no, no.

When you don't get enough sleep, it disrupts your hormones. These hormones will send signals to your brain to eat more, not because you're hungry, but because you didn't get enough sleep. Also, when you don't get enough sleep, you'll be tempted to skip exercise because, you guessed it, you're tired. Eating more and exercising less is a bad combination for fat loss.

Another way we can lose fat is through the proper consumption of water. Since your body is composed of 60 percent water, it is the basis for every chemical reaction that takes place, including burning fat. Water ensures our nutrients get digested properly; hence, it helps our organs function properly. You need your organs to function properly to lose fat.

For example, the kidney's job is to remove waste and extra water from your blood. If your kidneys do not remove this waste, the waste will build up in the blood and damage your body. Your kidneys need plenty of water to do this job efficiently. If your kidneys can't do this job entirely, your liver will assist in the process since it provides the body with energy. It does this by taking stored fat and turning it into energy that you can use. If you slow the process down, you slow down fat loss.

Drinking water and staying hydrated also plays another role in fat loss. It is estimated that up to 75 percent of Americans fall short of the 10 daily cups of water prescribed by the Institute of Medicine. This puts most people in the U.S in a chronic state of dehydration. If you are dehydrated, your muscles, which are made up of 70 percent water, won't function efficiently. Thus, it's impossible to maximize exercise if you're dehydrated. In fact, you'll probably just make the problem worse.

Consuming water also causes you to eat less. Yes, if you eat less, it's easier to create a caloric deficit necessary to lose fat. A recent study in the *Journal of Obesity* found that drinking 16 ounces of water before meals lead to additional weight loss. In this 12-week study of 84 adults with obesity, everyone was given general weight loss advice then assigned to one of two groups. One group was told to drink about 16 ounces of water thirty minutes before meals while the other group was told to simply imagine their stomachs were full before meals. The group that consumed water before meals lost about three more pounds than the group who merely imagined their stomachs full prior to eating meals.

Additionally, water serves as a substitute for juice, soda, and other high-calorie beverages. A switch to a healthy, zero-calorie beverage verses a high-calorie; high-sugar beverage has a direct impact on fat loss. Let's assume you drink five Cokes a week, that's 900 calories a week or 3,600 calories a month. Remember, a pound equals 3,500 calories.

The last way we can lose fat is through stress management. According to the American Psychological Association, weight loss is never successful if you remain burdened by stress and other negative feelings. Managing your stress is imperative if you're going to lose fat. For one, stress causes you to lose sleep. We just discussed the impact of getting too little sleep. Additionally if you're stressed, you're more likely to eat. Unfortunately, when people are stressed, they don't run to the salad bar, more than likely, it's to the dessert table.

When we're stressed, our body releases the cortisol hormone. Elevated cortisol levels increase the accumulation of abdominal fat. Just the opposite of your goal. Cortisol negatively affects fat loss by screwing up your hunger hormones, particularly Ghrelin and Leptin. Leptin helps to control your appetite while Ghrelin increases your appetite. When you are overly stressed, Leptin levels drop and Ghrelin levels increase making you hungrier. That's right, that's a double enemy to fat loss.

When you're stressed, it's difficult to maintain the caloric deficit needed for fat loss. Chronic stress makes fat loss impossible. If you intend to lose fat, stress management must be a part of your daily activities, like eating and exercising. We'll talk about stress management in chapter 12.

Now that you know how fat is lost, it's time to go back to the scale. Go stand on your scale.

Really ... go stand on your scale, and answer the following questions:

- Does the scale tell you if you ate at a calorie deficit today?
- Does it tell you if the exercise you did today was effective?
- Does it tell if you slept enough to burn calories and revive your body?
- Does it tell if you consumed enough water?
- Does it tell you how well you managed your stress?

The answer is no, no, no, no, and no. Get off the scale and don't get on it again, until after you have completed this program. Seriously. If you're one of those people who weigh themselves serially, give the scale to a friend across town. From now on, you'll use a scale that supports your goal of fat loss. A much more productive scale— *ThePerfectScale.*

Chapter 5—A New Scale

As with the old diet plan, your old method of measuring your success—getting on the scale—isn't productive. You bust your butt all week, you get on the scale, and there it is—the same weight as last week or maybe you're down a pound or two. I've seen this happen to so many clients. When it happens, their mood changes, and they're not as confident in their weight loss plan. Even worse, their motivation starts to disappear. All it takes is another week of little to no weight loss, or a stressful event, or any other reason to eat tasty, fatty, sugary food, and they're done. We, as a society, give too much power to the scale.

We need to stop giving power to the scale. About 15 years ago, I had a goal to weigh less than 200 pounds. I was eating great, working out religiously, lifting weights, and running. My body looked good, and I was just about beach ready. When I woke up one morning, I felt this was it: I had to be 200 pounds. I got on the scale and there it was—200.4 pounds. I did what any scale-possessed, goal-oriented person would do. I jumped off the scale, put on my shorts and running shoes, no shirt of course as I was beach ready, and I went for a run. I had to shed that four-tenths of a pound. I ran five miles. It was a July morning, so it was hot enough to work up a good sweat and burn some calories.

It was a great run. All I could think about was, "I did it. 200 pounds!" Goal attained. I couldn't wait to get back on that scale. I got back to the house, tossed the clothes, toweled off, started the shower, and jumped on the scale. There it was—201.6 pounds. You've got to be kidding me! How the heck did that happen? I didn't eat, and I burned calories, and I sweated. I wanted my reward. I wanted that 200 pounds.

Well, a lot goes on in your body once you start exercising and burning calories. So, I knew then and there that the scale didn't tell the whole story, and I needed to keep going and doing what I was doing, and then I would reach my 200-pound goal. Sure enough, later that week, I hit my goal.

But I was measuring the wrong thing—weight loss rather than fat loss. We are using the wrong tool to measure success. You need to measure everything that factors into your success. For example, let's say you have a goal to have a net worth of $1 million dollars. How do you measure that? You monitor every component related to net worth: your income, your expenses, your savings accounts, investments, your debt, property values, and any other relevant assets. You're going to measure all the things that will allow you to reach your goal. That's what *ThePerfectScale* does: measures all the factors.

I'm not saying that the scale is useless. It can be a good maintenance tool. However, your goal is not maintenance. Your goal is fat loss. With modern technology, there are scales claiming it can determine your body composition, in other words, how many pounds or percentage of muscle and fat your body contains. While fat is something that you want to measure, these scales aren't the most accurate, and using one every day is just as likely to result in frustration and discouragement, just like using the old scales.

At my studio, we use a high-end BIA (Bioelectrical impedance analysis) device to measure body fat. This device is very accurate and very expensive. We measure our clients monthly for fat loss and maintenance. Testing monthly provides an ample amount of time to see results. However, measuring monthly is too long for someone trying to lose fat now. Waiting until the end of the month to see results is like waiting until the end of the semester to see your grade when you're in college. There are opportunities along the way to see your grades and make improvements, just as there are opportunities to make adjustments in your eating and exercise routines to make improvements.

ThePerfectScale is ten times better than the scales used today. You can manually record your scale score on a piece of paper, or you can go to the app store and download the app for *ThePerfectScale*. Rather than measuring weight, my scale measures the important things. Every day it gives you an immediate, accurate score on your performance, providing prompt feedback as to where you need to focus to improve fat loss. That's right, you know exactly where to focus your attention and the areas that need improvement so you can get your body back in fat-burning mode.

The scale is a daily form, grading you on a ten-point scale. Just like in elementary school, your goal is to get an A every day, or 10 out of 10 points. If you get nine out of 10 points, you received an A minus for the day. Eight out of 10 is a B minus. Seven out of 10 is a C minus. Is eight out of 10 good? Yes, but nine or 10 out of 10 is better. Just like in school, you never want to get a C, D, or F. Unfortunately, many of you have been getting F's on a daily basis, and you don't even know it. If you had, you might have changed your behavior a long time ago.

The letter F hits home. It means failure, or, with my scale, weight gain or fat gain. The number on the traditional scale can be depressing, but it doesn't mean you failed; it doesn't have grades. But with *ThePerfectScale*, you can't hide from it since you receive immediate feedback in the form of a grade.

Here's how it works. On any given day, you can earn up to 10 points. The remainder of the book discusses how you earn these points in detail.

Nutrition (5 points)–You earn one point for each meal that you eat. Merely consuming food doesn't earn the point; there are some requirements for your meals. For now, just know you are expected to eat five times a day.

Exercise/Rest (1 point)–You earn one point per day for completing proper exercise outlined in this book. You are expected to exercise five days a week and rest two days. You actually earn a point for resting or taking time off from exercise.

Hydration (1 point)–You earn one point a day by drinking the appropriate amount of water. What's appropriate? Half your body weight in ounces. So, for example, if you weigh 200 pounds, then you need to drink 100 ounces of water daily.

Sleep (1 point)–You earn one point if you sleep for seven to nine hours. Sleep is very important to weight loss.

Stress Management (1 point)–You earn one point a day for managing your stress through meditation. To earn the point, you must meditate 10 to 15 minutes each day.

Planning (1 point)–You earn one point for planning your fat loss activities for the following day. Although it may not seem so, this is the most critical point and will ultimately determine your success. It's the most important point, and the old scale had no way of measuring it!!!

That's it. Your goal is to earn 10 points each day. Every day won't be perfect, but if you string together a series of good days, weeks, then months, you will not only feel and look better, but you will lose a significant amount of body fat. From here on out, we don't talk scale numbers, we talk points.

Let's do a quick test to see how you did yesterday. Answer these six questions. (Guide Activity)

1. How many meals did you eat? We are going to assume that they met the criteria to get a point even though they may not have. Give yourself a point for each meal. Let's say you ate three times yesterday, so you earned three points.

2. Did you exercise 30 to 45 minutes? If you didn't exercise yesterday but you exercise consistently, give yourself one point. If you don't exercise and you didn't exercise yesterday, give yourself a 0.

3. Did you drink half of your body weight in water? If so, give yourself one point.

4. How much sleep did you get? Give yourself one point if you slept between seven and nine hours.

5. Did you meditate or manage your stress? If not, give yourself a 0. If so, give yourself one point.

6. Did you plan your food, your exercise, and your stress management time for today? If you planned all three

of those, give yourself a point. If you did not plan what you're going to eat for lunch and dinner, when you're going to exercise, or when you're going to do your stress management, give yourself a 0.

Use Chart 1 to determine your score.

Chart 1. Your Score Card

Meals	_____ out of 5
Exercise	_____ out of 1
Hydration	_____ out of 1
Sleep	_____ out of 1
Stress Management	_____ out of 1
Planning	_____ out of 1

Based on this, your score is _____ out of 10

According to the scale, that's a _____

10	A
9	A-
8	B-
7	C-
6	D-
5	F

To be in fat loss mode, you need to score a nine or 10. (You can also be in fat loss mode with an eight, depending on how you earned the eight points.) Seven to eight points generally will put you in fat-maintenance mode. With six points or below, you will be in fat- gain or weight-gain mode.

At the end of the day, you can see exactly what you scored. You will have a grade, and you will also know exactly in what area you missed the mark. You can then target the area you need to work on to turn your body into a fat burning machine. Using the chart below, you can see your daily scores as well as your weekly score. Your goal is simply to earn 10 points a day or a minimum of 63 points for the week. To determine your score for the week, you will fill out a weekly chart. You can refer to Chart 2 as an example.

Chart 2. Example Weekly Score Card (Guide Activity)

	Monday	Tuesday	Wednesday	Thursday	Friday	Saturday	Sunday	Wkly Total	Wkly Avg
Meals	4	5	4	3	5	4	5	30	4.29
Exercise	1	1	1	1	1	1	1	7	1.00
Water	1	0	1	1	1	1	1	6	0.86
Stress Mgmt	1	1	1	1	0	1	1	6	0.86
Sleep	1	0	1	1	1	0	1	5	0.71
Planning	1	1	0	1	1	1	1	6	0.86
Daily Total	9	8	8	8	9	8	10	60	8.57

The Perfect Scale—The Ultimate Fat Loss System is that simple. Well, it's actually a little more complicated because there are negative points as well. We will discuss this in chapter 13.

Chapter 6—The Prerequisite

In the last chapter, I introduced you to the proper tool to measure and monitor your fat loss effort. Before we get into greater detail on the specifics of how you earn your points and why we are measuring these categories, we need to address a category not on the scale: you must change the way you think. You can't have success without changing this first.

I hope this book so far has enlightened you on fat loss and is starting to change how you will approach fat loss this time around. But that slight change, however, is not enough. A little change here or there is not enough. If you're going to pursue fat loss, you need to change the way you think, period.

I'll give you the information you need to implement to lose fat, but first, you need to change the way you think. Here's the first thing you need to know. Everyone's behavior fits into one of three categories.

1. You are eating and living to gain fat/weight.
2. You are eating and living to maintain your fat/weight.
3. You are eating and living to lose fat/weight.

Based on your behaviors, you fit into one of these three categories. The majority of the country is eating and living to gain fat/weight; thus, we are predominately an overweight or obese country. The facts support this.

Consider that, at this time in America, there are more overweight people than there are underweight people. Look back at the obesity charts in Chapter 2. What you see is a large group in the "eating and living to gain fat/weight category". Unfortunately, many people think they are in the maintenance category, but they are really in the gaining fat/weight gain category. As discussed previously, 90 percent of the people who lose weight put it back on. Only a small percentage of people are in the fat loss category. When people make an effort to lose fat/weight, they, unfortunately, don't change the way they think. They temporarily implement some diet or exercise routine and go back to their old habits and gain more fat/weight.

The mental change you need to make starts with your thinking. Your focus needs to be on fat loss, and the pursuit of fat loss. Once you lose the fat, then you change your focus to one of maintenance. When you're in fat loss mode, you can't live or operate the way you do now. Accept that you have been living a lifestyle of fat/weight gain that will rob you of your health, disable you with disease, and ultimately send you to an early grave.

Fat loss looks and lives nothing like that; it's just the opposite. Fat loss gives you health and quality of life. It prevents disease, and it ultimately prolongs health, thus life. If this is what you want, start thinking and behaving differently. Again, I will provide you with the information to behave differently, but you will have to do the thinking. I can't think for you. If you follow the plan, I guarantee fat loss and all the benefits that come with it. However, you have to guarantee me that you will think differently and align your thoughts with fat loss.

What does that mean? Think about a single person. They have the freedom and flexibility, the availability, to do just about anything. They have no commitments; if they want to, they can stay out all night. They have time to spend with friends, to go out on dates, and live spontaneously. I would classify this as the fat/weight gain lifestyle, if we were relating it to fat loss. Yes, fat/weight gain is like being single in that you have the freedom to eat and drink whatever and whenever you want. Yes, I know the single people are generally healthy, that is a reflection of their age or desire to look good to snag someone!

Now let's look at someone who is married. Married folks are committed to the relationship. They choose their battles. They sometimes have to do things they don't want to. They are consistent in their behavior. They're home every night, unless traveling for work. They spend time with their friends now and then. They go on date nights with their spouse here and there. They understand that being married is a top priority, and they work hard at it every day. By analogy, this would be classified as a fat/weight loss lifestyle. Yes, fat loss is like marriage in that it takes a serious commitment. You must be consistent, make it a priority, work hard on it every day, do some things that you don't want to, and pass on some things that you want to do. You have to be accountable. *Yes, I know a lot of married people are overweight, which may be a reflection of their settled lifestyle.*

If you try to do the "single" thing, while you're trying to lose fat, it's an automatic fail. Now that you know fat loss is like a marriage in many ways, you need to change your mindset from a single person to someone who is married. If you understand this, and you're ready to make the change, **LET'S GO!**

Just a quick side note—you don't have to stay in this stage for life. Just until you lose the fat you desire. Then you don't go back to being single, you move on to dating. Dating I would classify as fat/weight maintenance. I will share the maintenance program with you in my next book AFTER you lose the fat. First things first.

Chapter 7 — Planning

He who fails to plan, is planning to fail.—Sir Winston Churchill

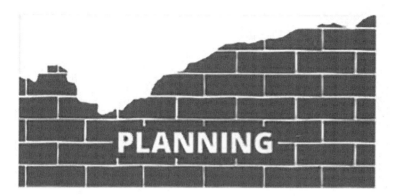

Planning, also sometimes referred to as forethought, is the process of thinking about and organizing the activities required to achieve a desired goal. In this case, your desired goal is fat loss. To plan for fat loss, you need to think about and organize all the activities required for fat loss: nutrition, exercise, hydration, rest, stress management, and planning.

Notice, planning is at the bottom of the diagram because planning is the foundation of fat loss. Without planning, your fat loss efforts will inevitably crumble and fail, just like a house built on a faulty foundation.

The foundation, in architectural terms, is the lowest load-bearing part of a building. It typically is below ground, and it supports the entire structure of a building. Would you build or move into a house that lacked a foundation to keep it solid, strong, and immovable? No. You want a solid foundation so your house can withstand storms, earthquakes, and any settling of the earth.

Planning is you laying the foundation for fat loss. If your fat loss efforts are going to stand the test of time; "storms," such as working late, holidays, travel; and "earthquakes" such as kids' schedules, late nights, parties, and so forth, you'd better plan. Planning is imperative to your success. You must plan every day. While you only receive one point for completing the requirements of planning, it's the most important component of *ThePerfectScale—The Ultimate Fat Loss System.* Just like it's the most important component of your house. You will not be successful if you don't plan. Each day, you'll need to set aside 15 minutes. Some days you'll need more. After you've established a routine, you'll be able to reduce the time spent planning.

You want to plan daily, so there are no surprises. You don't want to go to work without your lunch. You don't want to go without food because you're watching your child's soccer game. You don't want to leave your house in the morning without your workout clothes. You don't want to get so busy that you forget to meditate and address your stress. Failing to plan throws you off course. It's like a crack in your foundation. It will delay your progress, and possibly put an end to your fat loss efforts. It's impossible to get a 10 on the scale if you don't plan. When you don't plan, you lose, or should I say, gain fat/weight. You must plan the night before to ensure your success the following day.

In order to receive one point for planning, you must complete the following:

1. Pack any meals that you will not be eating at home. You should walk out the door with all the food you're going to eat until you return

2. Know what you will be ordering if you're eating out. I'll talk about this later on in the book

3. Know your workout time and have your workout clothes packed

4. Know when and where stress management will take place

5. Know what you're having for dinner the following day

If you complete all of these requirements, then you earn one point. If you miss any of these, you do not earn the point.

Here are some shortcuts to help you.

1. Delegate. I love this one. My daughters are awesome at making lunches. They do it for me after dinner while also doing the dishes. Have others help you plan.

2. Pick two or three restaurants to go when eating out. Figure out how to eat healthy in those restaurants, picking one or two healthy meals, and eat only those meals every time you go out. If friends want to go out to eat with you, insist on going to your restaurant. After you've completed the 12-week program, you can go to their restaurant.

3. If you must go to a "foreign restaurant," research online ahead of time and decide what you're going to eat. Don't review the menu once you get there. Make your decision ahead of time.

4. Handle stress management in the same place and time every day. I've created a nice space in my home where I meditate daily. You should do the same. If I can't do it at home because of my schedule, I have a couple of backup locations. If you're going to be away from your home, plan when and where you will meditate.

5. Put aside your workout clothes after you finish doing the laundry. There's no need to put them in a drawer. Put them in an additional gym bag and leave them in your car.

6. Plan your meals out for the week before you go grocery shopping.

7. Cook in batches/bulk a couple of times a week so you don't have to cook on a daily basis.

Chapter 8—Nutrition

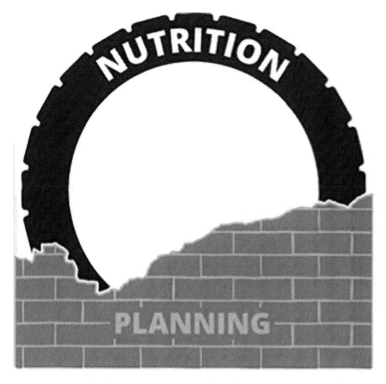

Just a quick review. First, in order to lose fat, you must change the way you think. The first step is planning how you will meet your goals. This planning is your foundation for fat loss and the most important daily point on *ThePerfectScale—The Ultimate Fat Loss System*. Now, let's turn our attention to nutrition.

Nutrition is the biggest component of fat loss; hence, it's the wheel in the fat loss diagram that gets and keeps fat loss in motion. It accounts for five, half of the points, on the 10-point scale. When practicing proper nutrition and eating the right amounts and types of food, you will lose body fat. What are the right types of food? You'll find the list in your guide.

Let's start with the basics. Eating for fat loss isn't the most fun. It's not fun like Chicken Parmesan or a juicy cheeseburger or chocolate cake. However, eating for fat loss isn't bad either. In fact, it's rewarding because every time you eat, you know you're eating to become healthy. That is the original purpose for food: for you to stay healthy. So don't complain about being bored or your lack of choices. Remember you're married (committed to his plan), so we'll find a way to spice it up, preventing you from boredom.

How much food should you eat? Go back to Chapter 4 or the calculation you did in your guide. If you did not do it, do it now to determine how many calories you should be consuming for fat loss.

Now is a good time to address a few important and often misleading statements I hear about fat/weight loss.

- "Calories in and calories out don't matter or work." Quick question. Did you gain weight by eating less and moving more? Of course not, it was from eating too much and moving too little. So, calories in (how much you eat) and calories out (how much you move) do matter.

- "Calorie counting is too hard and unnecessary." Really? If we understood how many calories were in our food, then maybe, just maybe, we wouldn't overeat! If we knew how many calories we were supposed to eat, we would learn a simple skill that we could use for the rest of our life to help us maintain our health!!! Don't be fooled by this nonsense. I'm not saying you need to memorize calorie charts or run to a food log and plug in your food intake every day; that's ridiculous. By simply following the meal plan, you will learn portion sizes, calories, and macronutrients. This will help you in maintenance and will make sure that you NEVER have to lose weight again. We go to school for 12 years, then many of us go to college. We work, take care of children, and yet, it's too hard to understand the makeup of the food we're eating! Give me a break!!

- "A calorie is a calorie." That isn't correct, either. According to the *Cambridge Academic Dictionary*, a calorie is a unit used in measuring the amount of energy food provides when eaten and digested. The calories in our food come from three macronutrients—protein, carbohydrates, and fats. One hundred calories of protein is not the same as 100 calories of carbohydrates. They may weigh the same amount, but they are not the same. They serve completely different purposes in our body. That's like saying one 200-pound body equals another 200-pound body. Not if one body has 180 pounds of muscle and 20 pounds of fat, compared to a body which has 100 pounds of muscle and 100 pounds of fat. They may weigh the same, but clearly, they are not the same and nor do they look the same.

Now that I've cleared up any misconceptions about calories and fat loss, let's dive into the structure of *ThePerfectScale—The Ultimate Fat Loss System* nutrition program.

Let's start with a breakdown of these three macronutrients—protein, carbohydrates, and fats—and examine the role that each plays in our body.

Table 1. The Three Macronutrients

Protein	
Proteins are the most abundant molecule in the body after water. Since they are responsible for every task of cellular life and cell replication, they can be found in all cells of the body. Additionally, they are responsible for many processes in the body and are required for the structure, function, and regulation of the body's tissues and organs. In fact muscle, organs, and connective tissue are comprised of protein. Protein is needed for body growth and maintenance. You must consume protein every day because your body does not have a way to store it. It can be used for energy if necessary.	Complete Proteins (Provide all of the essential amino acids) • Meat • Seafood • Dairy • Eggs Incomplete Proteins (Provide some of the essential amino acids) • Whole grains • Nuts • Legumes • Beans • Lentils

Carbohydrates	Simple Carbohydrates
Carbohydrates are the most efficient source of energy for fuel, providing energy to all cells of the body. Carbohydrates break down into glucose, which is our body and brains primary source of energy. Proper carbohydrate intake allows proteins to be used for tissue building and maintenance rather than energy. Additionally, carbohydrates also aid digestion by providing fiber which is essential for proper intestinal health. Fiber also helps lower cholesterol and decrease the risk of heart disease. However, not all carbohydrates are the same: they can be simple (like sugars), providing the body with quick energy; or complex (starches with fiber), providing sustained energy.	• Fruit • Dairy • Sugars • Honey • Baked goods • Candy Complex Carbohydrates • Whole grains • Brown Rice • Quinoa • Oats • Lentils • Leafy Green Vegetables • Sweet Potato
Fat	Monounsaturated and Polyunsaturated Fats
Fats, essential for the proper functioning of the body, help brain development, maintain core body temperature, cushion organs, control inflammation, act as a backup energy source when carbs are not available, and help absorb certain nutrients. Vitamins A, D, E, and K all rely on fat for absorption and storage. Your body can't make fat. Therefore, you must consume it every day. However, you want to ensure you consume more healthy fat. The healthy fats (good for your heart) are monounsaturated and polyunsaturated fats. The unhealthy fats (raise Low density lipoprotein— LDL) are saturated and trans fats.	• Vegetable oils • Nuts • Avocados • Salmon • Olive oil • Trout • Sardines • Seeds Saturated and Trans Fats • Processed Meat • Animal based products • Whole milk dairy products • Processed junk foods

Now that you understand the role of each, let's talk about how much to consume of each. *ThePerfectScale—The Ultimate Fat Loss System* meal plan calls for a 40/30/30 ratio. That is 40 percent of your calories will come from protein, 30 percent of your calories will come from carbohydrates, and 30 percent of your calories will come from fat. Here is a quick example. Let's say the calories needed for you to create a caloric deficit so that you burn fat are 1,500. We multiply that by the percentages to get the calories needed for each nutrient. See below.

1,500 X .40 = 600 calories of protein

1,500 X .30 = 450 calories of carbohydrates

1,500 X .30 = 450 calories of fat

We now need to take that one step further: calculate grams of each of the macronutrients. You need to know that a gram of carbohydrates and a gram of protein contain four calories while a gram of fat contains nine calories. We then divide the total calories by the calories per gram to get the grams needed. See below.

600 calories of protein ÷ 4 calories per gram = 150 grams of protein

450 calories of carbohydrates ÷ 4 calories per gram = 112.5 grams of carbohydrates

450 calories of fat ÷ 9 calories per gram = 50 grams of fat

This calculation demonstrates how many grams of each macronutrient you'll need each day. In this example, this person should intake 150 grams of protein, 112.5 grams of carbohydrates, and 50 grams of fat daily. Here's where it gets tough. You probably don't have the time or skills to create a meal plan that balances the calories and macronutrients. It would take a long time to calculate this. I know this for a fact because I use to do it for my clients manually. To assist you, I've created a meal plan at 1,250, 1,500, and 2,000 calories. You will find them in the guide. These are guidelines, not absolutes. You can play with them, make substitutions, and work the math until you get it right.

The provided meal plan fits the *ThePerfectScale—The Ultimate Fat Loss System* guidelines. DO NOT MAKE CHANGES to the macronutrient numbers. You can exchange the foods but not the macronutrients. It's been proven. Don't say it's too many calories and cut them yourself. You won't get the results. Don't say it's too many carbohydrates and cut them yourself. You won't get the same results. There is scientific reasoning behind the 40/30/30 ratio.

Remember that I mentioned that on this program, a person will not only lose fat but add muscle? You need muscle because once you're off the program and begin eating other foods; your body will be capable of metabolizing those other foods much better. To gain muscle, a person needs what's referred to as a one-to-one ratio. That is one gram of protein to one pound of body weight. The 40/30/30 ratio ensures that you get enough protein to build muscle. The 30 percent carbohydrates ensure that you have enough energy to get through the day and to exercise at a moderate to high intensity. The 30 percent fat requirement of the ratio makes sure your organs and brains function properly. So, don't screw this up! Stick to the 40/30/30 ratio. Got it?

ZIGZAG CALORIE APPROACH

Now that we've determined how many calories you need and what it looks like in terms of percentages, 40% protein, 30% carbohydrates, and 30% fat, it's time to introduce you to the zigzag calorie approach. This is also known as calorie shifting. This approach means you will fluctuate the number of calories you consume from day to day. There are several benefits to this, which I will explain shortly, but first let me explain how it's incorporated into *ThePerfectScale—The Ultimate Fat Loss System*. The meal plans call for a low/low/high calorie structure.

This means you will consume a low number of calories on days one and two, and a higher number of calories on day three. By low, I mean the number of calories you calculated for fat loss. This is considered low because its fewer calories than you need to maintain your current weight. You will consume this number of calories two days in a row. On the third day, you will consume an additional 250 to 500 calories.

Table 2. Zigzag Meal Plan based on calories

1,250 Calorie Meal Plan	1,500 Calorie Meal Plan	2,000 Calorie Meal Plan
Day 1–1,250 calories	Day 1–1,500 calories	Day 1–2,000 calories
Day 2–1,250 calories	Day 2–1,500 calories	Day 2–2,000 calories
Day 3–1,500 calories	Day 3–1,900 calories	Day 3–2,500 calories

After you consume the high day calories, 1,500, 1,900, or 2,500 respectively, you go back down to your fat burning number of 1,250, 1,500, 2,000 calories, respectively, for the next two days before bouncing back up to 1500, 1,900, or 2,500. See the example below.

Day 4–1,250 calories	Day 4–1,500 calories	Day 4–2,000 calories
Day 5–1,250 calories	Day 5–1,500 calories	Day 5–2,000 calories
Day 6–1,500 calories	Day 6–1,900 calories	Day 6–2,500 calories
Day 7–1,250 calories	Day 7–1,500 calories	Day 7–2,000 calories
Day 8–1,250 calories	Day 8–1,500 calories	Day 8–2,000 calories
Day 9–1,500 calories	Day 9–1,900 calories	Day 9–2,500 calories

As a society, we live differently on the weekends. Often time's clients find it easier for planning purposes to stick to the low calorie meal plan throughout the week and bump it up on the weekends. This is fine.

Table 3. Zigzagging on Weekends Meal Plan

1,250 Calorie Meal Plan	1,500 Calorie Meal Plan	2,000 Calorie Meal Plan
Monday–1,250 calories	Monday–1,500 calories	Monday–2,000 calories
Tuesday–1,250 calories	Tuesday- 1,500 calories	Tuesday–2,000 calories
Wednesday–1,250 calories	Wednesday–1,500 calories	Wednesday- 2,000 calories
Thursday–1,250 calories	Thursday–1,500 calories	Thursday–2,000 calories
Friday–1,500 calories	Friday–1,900 calories	Friday–2,500 calories
Saturday–1,500 calories	Saturday–1,900 calories	Saturday–2,500 calories
Sunday–1,250 calories	Sunday–1,500 calories	Sunday–2,000 calories
Monday–1,250 calories	Monday–1,500 calories	Monday–2,000 calories
Tuesday–1,250 calories	Tuesday–1,500 calories	Tuesday–2,000 calories

You're probably thinking this is a great deal of work, but it's not. There are sample meal plans at the back of the book and your guide which show how to incorporate the increase in calories. On another note, the high day is NOT to be interpreted as an eat-whatever-you-want or cheat day. This System does not encourage that type of behavior. Who are you cheating? "Cheat day" is a body building diet term and does not fit with our program.

On the high day, you continue to eat foods in the program just more of them. Why do you need to eat more every third day? Keep reading. Here's a quick story, and then I'll explain.

A recent study that followed a group of winners from the show, *The Biggest Loser*, concluded that six years after the show ended, 13 of 14 contestants in the study had regained a significant amount of weight. Four of them are heavier than they were before the show began! The story I want to share is about the 2009 winner, Danny Cahill. He lost 239 pounds on the show while dropping his weight from 430 to 191 pounds in just seven months! He had the biggest weight loss on the show, ever.

However, in a follow-up study, it was determined that because his metabolism has slowed, Cahill now burns 800 calories a day less than someone the same size. He's probably done permanent damage to his metabolism. This may haunt him for the rest of his life. Since winning the show, he's gained back over a hundred pounds. Can you imagine looking at someone who weighs the same as you, who can eat 800 more calories than you, and not gain any weight? 800 more calories!!!

This is one of the reasons why we fluctuate our calories. Our bodies want to be in the state of homeostasis. When we reduce our calories, over time, our body catches on and takes steps to ensure our survival. To conserve energy, hormones that regulate our metabolism in fat burning will decrease how much energy our body burns because it interprets this calorie reduction as a sign of famine or scarcity.

If you restrict calories for too long, you end up causing significant damage to your metabolism as in the case of Danny Cahill. With this system, your caloric deficit is not so low, and the exercise will not be so intense, so there isn't even a slight chance of this happening. However, the program is about speeding up your metabolism. Therefore, we put in the high days to prevent homeostasis and allow your body to stay in fat burning mode, thus preventing plateaus and stalling during the program.

The other benefits of the high day are as follows:

- It keeps your metabolism (BMR) revved up
- It supports lean tissue building, i.e., muscle maintenance and gain
- It prevents homeostasis by keeping your body guessing
- It prevents boredom, allows for variety, and makes you feel like you're not starving or dieting
- It increases your fat burning hormones
- You have more enjoyment and energy

Don't skip this step. Your fat loss may not be as dramatic or as fast initially as someone who goes on a restricted low-calorie diet, but in time, zigzagging or shifting your calories results in more fat loss, more muscle, and better results. Remember the tortoise and the hare? Don't be the hare! Follow the program and increase your calories every third day or on the weekends.

If you thoroughly reviewed the meal plan and the items on the food list you may have noticed that it is gluten and dairy free.

I always get the question why the meal plan is dairy and gluten free. Without going into too much detail, let's take them one at a time and see why they don't play into Perfect Scale—The Ultimate Fat loss plan. If you choose to include these items in your meal plan, you may slow your progress.

The USDA recommends 2-3 servings of dairy per day for bone health. They also recommend 6-11 servings of grains daily. However, these recommendations have come under scrutiny by many in the health and fitness world.

Dairy–Milk is a good source of calcium, potassium, vitamin D, and protein. Whole milk and many dairy products are also high in saturated fat. While dairy is not essential for humans, we have been told we need to consume it on a daily basis for our entire life. The funny thing is dairy wasn't even consumed until after the agricultural revolution. Prior to the agricultural revolution, humans only drank their mother's milk as infants. They didn't consume dairy as adults. The biological purpose of the cow's milk is to feed a rapidly growing calf since it is designed to provide all of the protein, micronutrients, and fatty acids that calves need to grow. By the time it is weaned, it weighs 8x its birth weight and NEVER drinks milk again. Milk is an excellent source of food and nutrition for a calf, but you are not a calf. No mammal drinks milk past infancy except for humans! We are the only species that consumes milk in adulthood, and the only species that consumes the milk of another animal! Our bodies weren't made to digest another animal's milk on a regular basis. Through time, we adopted the habit of drinking cow's milk. However, about 25% of the people in the US lose their ability to produce digestive lactase enzymes (lactose intolerance) after weaning (around 2 years old). 75% of the world's population is unable to break down lactose as well. Bottom line, the milk that was meant for you comes from your mother.

Milk used to be consumed unpasteurized or raw, but today it is a processed food. The current practice of homogenizing milk alters the milk's chemistry and actually increases the acidifying effects. Dairy cows are kept on sex hormones and pregnant for their entire lives in order to lactate year round and given antibiotics and synthetic hormones to increase milk production. You are consuming a lot of hormones and estrogen when you eat dairy. This includes organic milk. And as such, dairy products contribute ¼ to ½ of most people's dietary intake of dioxins, a term used to describe any highly toxic compound produced as the result of some manufacturing processes. Milk acidifies the body's pH which in turn triggers a biological correction. Calcium, which is largely stored in the bones, is an excellent acid neutralizer. Some believe that milk consumption leads to weaker bones because it leeches calcium from the bones. This is supported by statistics showing that countries with the lowest consumption of dairy products also have the lowest fracture incidence and countries with the highest rates of osteoporosis are the ones where people drink the most milk and have the most calcium in their diets.

The research on dairy has been very conflicting. Does it contribute to obesity, heart disease, type 2 diabetes, prostate cancer, bone density, Parkinson's disease, acne? It depends on who did the study! You can find research for and against dairy consumption, which I find very interesting.

If you have any sort of digestive problems, you should eliminate dairy and see how you feel. I can tell you I have not had a sinus infection or as much abdominal distress since eliminating dairy from my daily food intake. I currently eat it sparingly, which I recommend in the maintenance phase of the program. Everybody likes a little cheese and ice cream now and then.

Since dairy is not required for human survival, is a processed food, is full of hormones and antibiotics, and was never intended for human consumption, it is not on the meal plan. Consuming any dairy products during the program results in 0 points for the meal.

For those of you worried about how you will get enough calcium, I recommend dark green leafy vegetables. We absorb twice the amount of calcium when we eat veggies like kale, collard and turnip greens, broccoli, spinach and bok choy versus milk. Rice and almond milk are also alternatives to milk.

Gluten–As I mentioned earlier, the USDA recommends 6-11 servings of grains per day. That is probably why wheat is the single most cultivated crop worldwide. Most people eat it in every meal or at least a couple of times a day.

Wheat is an old food and has been around for over 10,000 years. However, over the last 60 years, the way we grow and process wheat has changed drastically. Almost all of the wheat eaten today is high yield dwarf wheat, which was developed by cross breeding and crude genetic manipulation in the 1950's and 1960's.

The proportion of gluten protein in modern wheat has increased enormously as a result of this hybridization. Research suggests that the human gut views gluten as a foreign invader against which it must mount an immune response.

In response to this dwarf wheat, many people have started eating Gluten Free foods and diets—excluding most grains. While going gluten free is only a requirement for those with Celiac disease, an autoimmune disease where the body reacts negatively to gluten because it damages the intestines, my program asks you to stay away from it since it is genetically modified. Celiac and gluten intolerance have risen four fold since the 1950's. Even with the increase, less than 1% of people are diagnosed with celiac disease. Gluten sensitivity may affect up to 3%-5% of the population.[1] To determine if you have Celiac disease, you will need to undergo a blood test and bowel biopsy. To determine if you have gluten intolerance, look for the following symptoms diarrhea, constipation, nausea and abdominal pain. If you experience any of these symptoms after consuming wheat or grains, you may want to consult your doctor and minimize those foods in your diet.

Along with introducing dwarf wheat, today's modern wheat is also processed differently. The modern steel mill roller is more efficient and results in lower production cost, but it causes the vital nutrients to be stripped and processed out. This refined wheat is not only nutrient deficient; it spikes your blood sugar when consumed.

Wheat has been genetically modified to increase its yield and reduce its cost. It looks nothing like the amber waves of grain referred to in "America the beautiful." It's more like a little dwarf wheat that is resistant to everything: Pest, droughts, and especially chemicals!!! Pure and simple it isn't food. It's a far cry from the wheat our grandparents ate. Because wheat is a processed food, raises blood sugar, can cause inflammation in the gut, and contains gluten, it is not included in the food list. Barley and rye have been excluded as well.

---

1   Samuel O. Igbinedio, Junaid Ansari, Anush Vasikaran, Felicity N. Gavins, Paul Jordan, Moheb Boktor, and Jonathan S. Alexander, "Non-celiac gluten sensitivity: All wheat attack is not celiac." *World Journal of Gastroenterolgy*23, no. 40 (October 28, 2017): 7201-210. Accessed December 2017. doi: 10.3748/wjg.v23.i40.7201.

ThePerfectScale—The Ultimate Fat Loss Program is gluten free. That means the nutrition program does not does not contain any bread, cakes, cereals, cookies, crackers, pastas, pies, fried foods, processed foods, whole wheat flour and white flour, barley, rye or processed meats. Beer is also excluded. That's right no beer, but wine and tequila are good! See chapter 13 regarding alcohol.

For grains and starches, we include oatmeal, buckwheat, millet, quinoa, and rice (various types) on the program.

Gluten-free products are all the rage now as their sales exceed $5 billion. However, please understand that just because foods are labeled gluten free, it doesn't make them healthy foods. Don't buy them unless they are fruits, vegetables, eggs, fresh meats, fish, chicken, beans, seeds nuts, and the grains previously mentioned.

In terms of *ThePerfectScale*, any meal eaten that includes gluten is 0 points. You can bring these foods back in during the maintenance stage.

While you do not get a point for it, if you are going to eat wheat, I recommend Stone-ground "whole meal" flour. It may be difficult to find and won't last as long as commercial produced flour.

If you would like to read more on wheat and grains, I recommend the following books, *Wheat Belly* by Dr. William Davis, *Grain Brain* by Dr. David Perlmutter, and *The No-Grain Diet* by Dr. Joseph Mercola.

In order to get one point for a meal, it must consist of or look very similar to what is on your meal plan in terms of calories and macronutrient breakdown. If you eat something that is not on the plan or skip a meal, you don't get the point. This shouldn't happen if you plan properly.

Tips:

- Go grocery shopping every week
- Cook in bulk. You don't need to cook everything for the week on Sunday and put it in 35 plastic containers. That's body building. You have a lot more flexibility on your meal plan.

However, it helps to cook enough food so that it last for a few days, so you don't have to cook every day

- Put snacks every place you go. (Car, office, gym bag). If you need to eat, you can quickly get to your food
- Plan your meals ahead of time. There is plenty of variety on this meal plan if you plan ahead
- Use protein shakes and bars when it's inconvenient to sit down and eat a meal
- Don't bring food into the house that is not on the plan
- Buy prepared foods. I buy a rotisserie chicken every week. They're available at most grocery stores, and it makes life easier. Just make sure what you purchase is included on your meal plan. Be careful and ask questions about preparation, if necessary.
- When eating out at restaurants, make sure your meal follows your meal plan

As a Certified Nutritional Fitness Specialist, I provide nutritional counseling. If you desire a custom plan that works for you, I recommend you purchase my custom nutritional counseling and coaching. It's much easier to lose fat when a plan is designed specifically for you, with foods you like and you have someone to guide you along the way. I guarantee results. You will find a discount code for my nutritional services in your guide. They can be purchased from my website, TheFitnessProfessor.com.

Chapter 9—Exercise

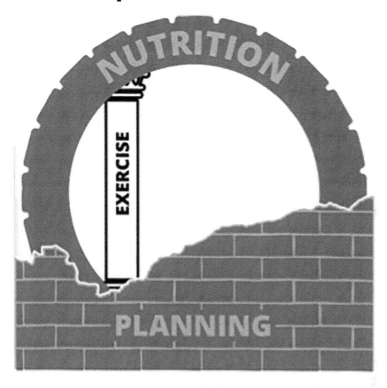

Let's clear the air on exercise: Exercise is not the best way to lose weight. I'm an exercise guy, and I can tell you from personal and professional experience as well as research, you do not lose a significant amount of weight or fat through exercise alone. According to research, the best way to lose weight is through proper nutrition, which is why it makes up half the points on the fat loss scale. Don't misunderstand me; exercise is important to fat loss and for your health. Exercise and nutrition go hand in hand like Batman and Robin, Venus and Serena, and peanut butter and jelly—on gluten free bread! Since they work so well together, it's the first spoke in the wheel of *ThePerfectScale—the Ultimate Fat Loss System* diagram.

The spoke for exercise counts as one point on *ThePerfectScale*. Exercise does help burn calories and increase your metabolism, so it does contribute to fat loss just not as much as nutrition. Nutrition is number one; exercise is number two. I like to call it Nexercise. ™ You will never be able to out-exercise a bad diet, but just like the dynamic duo of Michael Jordan and Scottie Pippen, combining exercise with good nutrition provides you with a dual edged sword that is guaranteed to be successful.

Let's talk about why exercise is number two. Total energy expenditure, TEE, is the number of calories burned by the human body in one day, adjusted to the amount of activity. Let's say you burn 2,500 calories with a basal metabolic rate of 1,750 calories (60-80 percent of your TEE). Then to break down the food you eat throughout the day requires 250 calories (10 percent of your TEE). You might expend 500 calories of energy during the day through physical activity (10-30 percent of your TEE). Therefore, when you exercise, you are only working on the 10 to 30 percent of your total energy expenditure, so you can make an impact, but it will be small. Visually, it would look like table 4.

Table 4. Total Energy Expenditure (TEE) = 2,500 calories

1750 Calories Basal Metabolic Rate	250 Calories Food Break Down	500 Calories Activity

Food, on the other hand, accounts for the entire amount of energy intake. Get that right, and you'll make a big impact.

Many don't lose weight while exercising because they tend to overeat or increase their food consumption when they exercise. It's the "I exercised today, so I can eat an extra slice of pizza" mentality, in other words, the Compensation Theory. Remember, I told you I ran two half-marathons and gained weight both times. I was expending a significant amount of calories in training, but I was also consuming too much food for weight loss.

Additionally, after exercising for extended periods of time, your body reacts by slowing down its basal metabolic rate, so you don't burn as much energy. That's what happened to the winners of *The Biggest Loser*. Excessive exercise is not a good thing. *ThePerfectScale—The Ultimate Fat Loss Program* calls for you to exercise only five days a week for 30 to 45 minutes and rest the other two. Don't exercise any more than this. The benefits do not outweigh the time spent, and you will not accelerate your results. In fact, you may increase your chances of getting injured. If this seems like a lot of exercise, don't worry, I recommend you reduce the amount and type of exercise you do after you lose the desired amount of fat and enter the maintenance phase.

You may be thinking, "If I don't lose a significant amount of weight exercising, then why bother at all. I'll just eat better; that's enough." I say, have you ever had fajitas? It's one of my favorites. I love the smell, the taste, and the sizzle. You can hear it as soon as it comes out of the kitchen. Can you imagine fajitas without the sizzle? They just wouldn't be the same, nor would they look or taste as good. Well, exercise is the sizzle. It makes eating right feel and look so much better, and the health benefits are endless, and I mean endless.

According to the Centers for Disease Control, regular physical activity is the most important thing you can do for your health. It can help control your weight, reduce the risk of cardiovascular disease, reduce the risk of Type 2 diabetes and metabolic syndrome, reduce the risk of some cancers, strengthen bones and muscles, and improve mental health and mood. Other benefits of exercise include:

- Improves one's ability to perform activities and can help prevent falls for older adults, by improving posture, balance and coordination
- Increases longevity
- Reduces blood pressure and triglyceride levels in your blood.
- Reduces the risk of stroke and heart attack
- Lowers the risk of developing cognitive impairment from Alzheimer's disease or dementia

- Helps control weight, combats health conditions, and boosts your level of energy
- Facilitates better sleep
- Puts the spark back into your sex life
- Reduces stress and increases relaxation
- Boosts happy chemicals and endorphins in your body
- Alleviates anxiety
- Improves self-confidence
- Sharpens memory
- Prevents cognitive decline
- Helps control addiction
- Increases energy levels
- Boosts your immune system not to mention the anti-aging qualities it provides by strengthening your heart
- Eases back pain

Remember, exercise and sound nutrition together, is the best medicine, and should be the first medicine you ever take. Now that I've got you sold on exercise, due to all those benefits, let's talk about the type of exercise you're going to be doing.

Alywn Cosgrove, the guru of fat loss and creator of the term metabolic resistance training, has reviewed extensive research on exercise and fat loss. He has created what he terms the hierarchy of fat loss training. In the hierarchy of fat loss training, you prioritize your exercise based on what is most efficient for fat loss and how much time you have available to exercise.

The hierarchy of fat loss training:

1. Metabolic resistance training
2. Non-traditional anaerobic interval training
3. Traditional interval training
4. Steady state high intensity aerobic training
5. Steady state low intensity aerobic training

He recommends number one, metabolic resistance training, and number two, non-traditional anaerobic interval training, for anyone pursuing fat loss with three to six hours to exercise per week. Number three, traditional interval training, is not recommended unless one has more than six hours a week to exercise. Number four, steady state high intensity aerobic training, requires you have more than eight hours to exercise a week. No one, according to Cosgrove, should pursue number five unless he or she can devote more than 10 hours a week to exercise.

A review of this shows why most people don't lose weight when they exercise. The majority of people begin with the least effective form of exercise for fat burning—aerobic training. This form of steady state training, for instance, getting on the treadmill and walking, running five miles per hour, or jumping on an elliptical machine is simply a waste of time—if you're trying to lose fat. This has been proven in numerous studies.

In one 12-month study, participants did aerobic training for 50 minutes, six days a week, for one year. The average total weight loss was only three and a half pounds, or three-tenths of a pound per month. That sucks. Over 15,000 minutes of exercise and only an average of three and one-half pounds were lost. Can you say ineffective? Walk into almost any gym, and the first thing you see is people on these machines, wasting their time. Why? Because they don't understand how to exercise for fat loss. Why doesn't the gym tell you that? They sell memberships not fat loss. Don't get me started on them!

What is metabolic resistance training? According to Alwyn Cosgrove, it's a modification of traditional resistance training to maximize fat loss by increasing the caloric burn during the activity and metabolic rate after the activity. The goal of metabolic resistance training is to work large muscle groups hard, frequently, and with enough intensity to create a metabolic disturbance for an after-burn that leaves your metabolism elevated for hours after the workout.

The after-burn, or excess post exercise oxygen consumption (EPOC), is the additional oxygen needed after exercise to return your metabolic rate back to pre-exercise levels. During EPOC, additional calories are burned. This is what makes this form of exercise better than aerobic training. This means that in order to maximize fat loss, you need to do metabolic resistance training, not Zumba, Yoga, Pilates, Hot Yoga, walking, elliptical, or whatever is the latest non-EPOC inducing exercise trend. After reaching your fat loss goal, you can bring some of these other forms of exercise back into your routine, but in terms of fat loss, you must recognize that they're a waste of time. Not that they're bad, but they're not the most effective and efficient type of exercise for fat loss.

Quick question: Would you bang in a nail with a screwdriver? A wrench? Pliers? Or a Hammer? You would use a hammer because it's the most effective and efficient tool for the job. That is what metabolic resistance training is: the best form of exercise for the job—fat loss. The other types of exercise are efficient tools for goals other than fat loss.

Follow *ThePerfectScale—The Ultimate Fat Loss System* workout routine and you'll be set. It includes metabolic resistance training, anaerobic interval training, strength training, and HIIT training. You may not be able to complete the workouts in their entirety initially, but within a short period of time, you will be completing it and progressing.

As always, get your doctor's approval before you start the workout regimen. Each workout consists of a warm up, exercise routine and a cool down. If you are not familiar with the exercises in the program, I suggest you do some research, buy my exercise DVD, or sign up for online training. I have included a written version of the program in the guide. The exercise program assumes you have access to a gym or fitness facility.

As you will see, it's a five-day exercise program. Each day you complete the exercise program, you earn a point. You also earn a point each for taking two days off during the week. Remember, rest is important. Do not exercise on your off days. That doesn't mean you sit on the couch all day, but don't exercise. I recommend you take a day off during the week and a day off on the weekend (For example, Thursday and Sunday). An exercise day on the weekend will prevent you from eating too much and sitting around. However, you base it on your work and life schedule. Just make sure you schedule five days of exercise per week.

In order to get a point for exercise, you must exercise properly, as prescribed, for 30 to 45 minutes. A boot camp class with weights can be substituted for the recommended workouts. Running on the treadmill or doing a butt and gut class doesn't count. You get 0 points for that. You can bring in alternative forms of exercise once you complete the program. If you exercise an additional day beyond what your program requires either four or five days, you don't get a point for that day, you get a 0. REST is very important.

Here are my recommendations in terms of exercise:

1. Work out at home. I highly recommend this. This will save you travel time to and from the exercise facility. That time could be your exercise time. Also, bad weather will never be an excuse not to exercise. If you have the equipment in your house, you will be able to workout at your convenience. If you don't already have exercise equipment in your home, you should get some. Exercise is the best medicine on the market. Do you have Advil, ibuprofen, Nyquil, or any other medicine in your medicine cabinet? If so, then you should have exercise equipment in your home, too. It's a small investment for a lifetime of benefits. You may need to purchase some equipment if you decide to do this. However, you don't need to buy an entire gym. I have included my recommendations for equipment in the guide.

2. Get a workout partner. This will help with support and accountability. Two is always better than one.

3. Hire a trainer. This is not required, especially if you buy the DVD or purchase online training, however, a trainer will move you through the exercises quickly, ensure proper form, give you a kick in the butt when you need it, and hold you accountable.

4. Set a specific time to exercise. Put it in your schedule like a doctor's appointment. Don't give this time up for anyone, not even your kids. Plan accordingly.

5. If, for some reason you don't exercise at home, find a gym that is not crowded so you won't be bothered and you can get to the equipment that you need. It is tough doing multiple exercises at a gym. When you move from one piece of equipment, someone will use or move it. If that's how you choose to exercise, good luck.

I recommend you purchase the in home workout DVD and workout from home. It will save you time but certain equipment is required. If you would like a more specific custom workout for your needs, go to TheFitnessProfessor.com and sign up for a custom program. My online training programs are inexpensive and take the guess work out of exercise. They will ensure that you progress, add muscle, and burn fat throughout the 12 weeks and beyond. You will save a lot of time and effort by using my programs or DVD. If you want to move the needle on your fitness level, sign up to work with me. I guarantee you results.

Chapter 10—Sleep

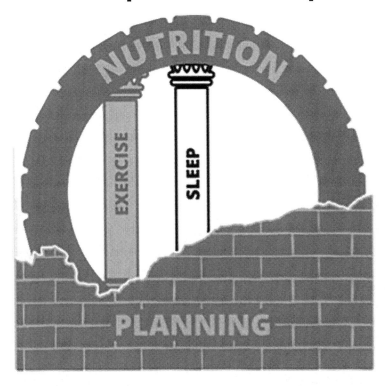

You're having a stellar day in terms of *ThePerfectScale*. You woke up, had a great breakfast, and went to the gym or to the basement to lift some weights. As you worked up a great sweat, you realized you're improving: You followed your meal plan all day, drinking plenty of water, went outside, got some fresh air, sat in your car and meditated for 15 minutes. All is well. You're racking up the points. After planning for the next day, the only thing left for a perfect day is a good night's rest. But first you decide to relax and watch the latest episode of *Game of Thrones*. You're a little worked up after watching it and not quite ready for bed, so you decide to check your email, maybe surf the web, or check Facebook.

Glancing at the clock, you realize it's midnight. Knowing you have to get up in six hours, you immediately go to bed, but you lay awake for 30 to 45 minutes before finally falling asleep. Guess what? You ruined your perfect day. Sure, you don't have a horrible score. You'll get nine out of ten points for the day, but your lack of sleep negates a lot of the hard work you did. It can get worse. Chances are you're going to eat bad food the next day and maybe you'll be too tired to exercise. Yes, sleep is that important. Sleep is as important to fat loss as nutrition and exercise. That point is worth repeating. Sleep is as important to fat loss as nutrition and exercise.

In fact, a consistent lack of sleep has been associated with diabetes, high blood pressure, and heart disease, all which have been on the rise for the past 40 years. Over that time, daily sleep duration in the United States has decreased by an hour and a half to two hours. The number of young adults sleeping less than seven hours has doubled to 37.1 percent. According to the CDC, 35% of Americans are sleep deprived. A recent Gallup poll showed that 40 percent of Americans said they get just six hours of sleep or less a night. It is also estimated that some 50 to 70 million Americans suffer from some type of sleep disorder.

Without proper sleep, your fat loss efforts will look like a dog chasing its tail. You can keep trying and trying, but you'll never get there, or if you do, you won't be there very long. Sleep is so important to fat loss that it's the second spoke in the nutrition wheel, counting for one point. Many people do not realize how sleep impacts their eating habits. There is such a strong correlation that sleep deprivation is now recognized as a risk factor for obesity. It is estimated that sleep deprived people consume about 300 to 500 more calories daily versus well-rested people because their sugar cravings and desire to eat high-carbohydrate junk food increases. Remember those obesity charts at the beginning of the book? Each decade we became heavier and heavier. Guess what? The amount of sleep we get also decreased significantly during that time.

So why is sleep so important? Sleep allows the body to repair and rejuvenate itself. Many other major restorative functions of the body occur during sleep—such as muscle growth, tissue repair, restorative functions, protein synthesis, and regulation of hormones, to name a few.

How does insufficient sleep affect your body? Basically, a lack of sleep contributes to weight gain due to two hormones that control your appetite, leptin and ghrelin. Leptin is produced in your fat cells and is responsible for controlling your appetite. It tells you when you're full. When you don't get adequate sleep, your body produces less leptin and lowers the level of leptin in your body. The less you have, the more you want to eat. The hormone, Ghrelin, on the other hand, is released by your stomach, and it stimulates hunger. When you don't get enough sleep, your body produces more ghrelin, which makes you hungrier. This is a vicious cycle that you will never beat. Your willpower is no match for this.

Since you feel hungrier, you will eat more, especially since a lack of sleep also increases your eating time. The less time you spend sleeping means the more time you are available to eat. It's simple math. The more time you have available to eat and the hormonal changes that accompany lack of sleep spell disaster. Usually this leads to late night eating and daytime snacking, causing weight gain, mainly fat gain, and muscle loss.

In addition to problems with your leptin and ghrelin, your cortisol levels rise. Cortisol is a stress hormone (discussed more in chapter 12). High cortisol levels result in increased fat storage and the inability to build muscle, resulting in a lower metabolism and activating an area of your brain that makes you want food. A combination of low leptin (police), extra ghrelin (bad guys), and an increase of cortisol (more bad guys), triggers a hunger cycle that even food can't satisfy, at least healthy food can't. If you eat healthy under these circumstances, you will still be hungry and unsatisfied after you've eaten.

Table 5. Impact of Sleep on Cortisol, Leptin and Ghrelin.

Adequate Nights Rest	Inadequate Nights Rest
Cortisol–Normal	Cortisol–Increase fat storage ↑
Ghrelin–Normal	Ghrelin–Increase in hunger ↑
Leptin–Normal	Leptin–Decreases appetite control ↓

It gets worse yet. When you don't get enough sleep, you reduce your insulin sensitivity and your production of growth hormones. Without the needed insulin, you decrease your glucose tolerance, which means you're more likely to store food as fat. This is also a path to diabetes. Not only do you store more fat, but you don't build muscle without your growth hormones. Growth hormones support cell rejuvenation, reproduction, and growth. This is a terrible chain of events that all started with that decision to watch *Game of Thrones* and not get a minimum of seven hours of sleep.

Clearly, you can see lack of sleep can lead to obesity. No sleep equals weight gain.

Along with impacting your eating habits, fat intake, and ability to build muscle, lack of sleep decreases your chance of exercise. Most people already find it difficult to exercise. If you think you're going to exercise when you're tired, forget it. It's hard to exercise when you are not very alert. All day you operate in a state of brain fog. Most people address this with coffee, sugary beverages, or the snack machine. Your body needs energy to cover for the lack of sleep, and these provide it quickly and conveniently. The only problem is they make you fat and sick.

If all of this wasn't bad enough, lack of sleep also decreases your immune function. Again, sleep is the opportunity for your body to heal and rejuvenate itself. If you don't allow your body proper time to heal and continue making impossible demands, you will ultimately compromise your immune system, making you susceptible to illness. Try losing fat while sick. Good luck with that. This spells fatigue and irritability. You'll become a cranky McCrank monster. Not getting enough sleep makes you tired, which makes you stressed and difficult to deal with. Reducing your caloric intake alone does enough sometimes to tip your mood in the wrong direction. Try not getting enough sleep at the same time, and people won't want to be around you.

If I haven't convinced you to sleep at least seven hours yet, I can tell you from my personal experience that I lived a sleep deprived life for several years, maybe a decade. It wasn't until I conducted the research for this book that I fully became convinced of the damage I had caused. When I went through the 12-week program, I changed my bedtime to 10 p.m. I usually wake at 5 a.m. and I could tell a difference immediately. My cravings were gone, I felt alert and happier, and it was easier to drop weight compared to previous attempts. If you get one thing out of this book, start sleeping. I've now made it my best friend and secret weapon for keeping the fat off. From time to time, I may not get my seven hours, but I get right back on track, ASAP.

Below are some interesting statistics on sleep.

- A study from the University of Chicago compared the weight loss results for two groups. While they both ate the same amount of calories, one group slept eight and a half hours per night and the other slept for five and a half hours per night. Even though both groups lost six and a half pounds, the well-rested group lost more fat. The sleep-deprived group's weight loss only comprised of 25 percent fat loss. This supports two studies, the first from the *American Journal of Clinical Nutrition*, which found that normal sleepers have a higher metabolism than those who don't get adequate sleep. The second from scientists in Brazil who found that a lack of sleep decreases protein synthesis, which causes muscle loss. Again, refer to earlier in the book when we talked about the importance of muscle. We never want to lose muscle, just fat.

- In the largest analysis of over 68,000 women, aged 45 to 65, referred to as the *Nurses' Health Study*, researchers followed women for 16 years, asking about their weight, sleep habits, diet, and other lifestyle aspects. At the start of the study, all of the women were healthy. None were obese. Just 16 years later, women who slept five hours or less per night had a 15 percent higher risk of becoming obese compared to the women who slept seven hours per night. Short sleepers also had added 30 pounds over the course of the study compared to women who got seven hours of sleep per night!!!

In order to get a point for sleeping, you must sleep between seven and nine hours. If you wake up in the middle of the night to use the bathroom, that time does not count against your sleeping time. However, if you wake up for more than 20 minutes after you initially fall asleep, that time needs to be subtracted from your final sleep time. Seven or more hours is your goal. If you sleep less than seven, then you won't get the point. If you sleep more than nine hours, you don't get a point because weight gain is also associated with sleeping more than nine hours. I didn't spend much time discussing it because that doesn't seem to be a problem for most Americans. However, if you sleep more than nine hours, set an alarm and get up between eight to nine hours after falling asleep.

Here are some tips to help you sleep better.

- Develop a bedtime routine. It should include going to bed and waking at a consistent time each day
- Turn off your technology an hour or two before going to bed, preferably two to three hours before turning in
- Do relaxing activities before bedtime. Read, take a bath, meditate, etc.
- Avoid caffeine and alcohol before bedtime
- Finish exercising and eating several hours before bedtime
- Have sex before going to bed. It promotes sleep. I call it a natural sleeping pill
- Create a sleep atmosphere in your bedroom. It should be quiet, dark, relaxing, and cool
- Get the animals out of your bed
- Supplement with Sleepytime tea, calcium, and magnesium or melatonin
- See a medical professional if you have chronic sleep issues

Chapter 11—Hydration

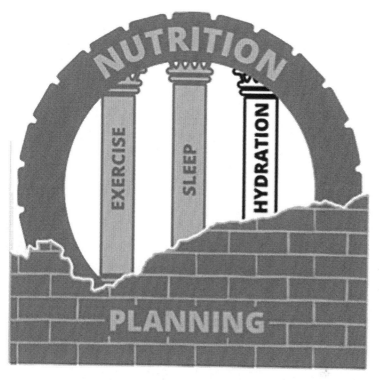

Hydration, the third spoke in the nutrition wheel, supports the wheel of nutrition and overall health while contributing to your fat loss efforts. You're probably thinking what does water have to do with fat loss? I am sure you have heard or read previously that you should drink six to eight glasses of water a day. I'll get to that in a moment, but first I want to emphasize the importance of water to your life. That's right, your life. Not your health, but your life. The average human will not survive without consuming water for three to four days. Since a human can survive much longer without food, Mahatma Gandhi survived 21 days fasting—more than once, water is more important than food.

If water is so important to your survival, then it's going to be important to your fat loss. In fact, two-thirds of your body is water. We need water to carry nutrients and oxygen throughout our body, help control our body temperature, digest our food, maintain the body's fluid balance, eliminate waste, lubricate our joints, and help our cells grow and reproduce. Additional benefits of drinking water include flushing out toxins, helping maintain regular bowel movements, improving skin complexion, improving mood, preventing cramps, and helping you think more clearly. It's even a headache remedy and cheaper than most beverages because it's free!

It does all this for your body, and it helps you lose weight. Currently, people in the US drink soft drinks more than water. No wonder obesity and diabetes are on the rise. A switch from soft drinks to water alone would make a significant impact on our nation's health. While soft drink sales are currently on the decline, the elimination of them is truly the answer. Nowhere on this program is there a place for soft drinks. Drinking your calories is simply a weight gain behavior, and that's not our goal. Water is calorie-free: it contains no protein, no carbs, no fat, and no sugar. By simply replacing high calorie, high sugar beverages with water, you automatically reduce your caloric intake.

Epidemiological studies suggest that calorie intake is significantly lower, nine percent or 194 calories, in water drinkers compared to non-water drinkers. I'll drink to that! As I mentioned previously, in a study of 84 middle-aged overweight and obese participants, those who drank 16 ounces of water 30 minutes before their meals compared to those who didn't lost three more pounds. Those who drank 16 ounces before every meal lost nine pounds over the 12 week experiment. Another study concluded that people who drank two cups of water prior to a meal ate between 75–90 fewer calories during that meal.

Water fills your stomach and helps you feel satisfied, which limits your desire to drink or eat unhealthy alternatives. You also need water to perform during exercise. Being dehydrated will prevent you from exercising at maximum capacity, which not only negatively impacts your results, but also your caloric and fat burning outcomes. Drinking water increases the amount of calories you burn by increasing your resting metabolic rate (RMR). While this increase is minimal, any increase in your RMR is welcomed.

One note, on this program, you may consume more protein than you may be used to, causing your kidneys to work harder to process this protein. To avoid health problems, you need to drink water since it helps your kidneys remove waste products and excess fluid from the body.

What's needed to get a point? How much water should you drink? The health community recommends six to eight cups of water daily. This is a general recommendation, which needs to be adjusted for activity, exercise level, exercise intensity, duration of exercise, health conditions, pregnancy, breast feeding, and your environment.

To receive the point for water, you need to drink half of your bodyweight in ounces of water. For example, if you are 200 pounds, we divide your weight in half, 200 divided by two equals 100. You need to consume 100 ounces of water daily. That is your goal. If you consume 80 ounces of water, you've done a good job, but you do not get the point. Coffee and alcohol are diuretics, so they do not count towards your water goal. You can drink as much coffee as you like on this program although I would limit it to no more than two cups a day, especially if you're having problems sleeping. In terms of alcohol, it's not recommended and has an adverse effect on your daily score (see chapter 13 for the negatives).

Yes, you can get water by consuming fruit and vegetables. However, most of your fluid needs are met through water and other beverages you drink. We are not going to count fluids from fruits and vegetables because it's entirely too difficult to measure and unnecessary. Consider any water consumed through the consumption of fruit and vegetables to be a bonus.

How do you know if you're properly hydrated? You should not feel thirsty, your urine should be colorless or light yellow, and you should be urinating six to eight cups of water regularly. No need to measure this unless you really think you have a health problem.

Here are some tips to help you consume half your bodyweight in ounces of water daily.

- If you currently are not drinking much water, build up to your goal slowly. You should be able to reach it within a week or two
- Water and tea count towards your daily goal, so drink a large cup or two of green tea daily
- Buy a water bottle and fill it up to track your consumption. This makes it easy
- Keep your water bottle handy so drinking is convenient
- Consume water before, during, and after your workouts
- Consume water before, during, and after a meal
- Cut off drinking at a certain time in the evening, so you aren't waking up in the middle of the night to go to the bathroom
- If you're going to drink protein shakes, the water in your protein shake counts towards your daily goal
- Start the day off drinking water. You may add lime or lemon to your water for taste, but do not add sweeteners
- I do not recommend calorie-free flavor unless it's natural and doesn't contain artificial sweeteners

Chapter 12—Stress Management

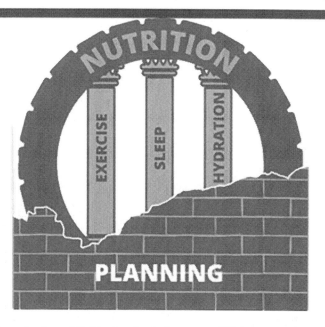

STRESS MANAGEMENT

Let's take a look at *ThePerfectScale* diagram. We've just about walked through the entire diagram, but let's do a quick review. At the bottom is the foundation—planning. On top of the foundation is the house or the wheel of nutrition. The wheel of nutrition is supported by three pillars: exercise, sleep, and hydration. At the top of the diagram is the roof representing stress management. Very few, if any, weight loss programs ever discuss stress management.

I'm here to tell you that stress will blow the roof off your fat loss goals and make you fat, sick, and overwhelmed. It is at the top of the diagram because any pressure on either end of the stress bar will send the wheel of nutrition and its pillars rolling off its foundation.

If you are going to try to lose fat, as discussed earlier, it takes time—12 weeks or more. Time equals consistency. In order to be consistent with your efforts, you must have your stress under control. Therefore, a stress management aspect has to be included in your weight loss regimen. If stress management isn't part of your weight loss plan, you're destined for failure.

Why? Because stress wreaks havoc on your body, and it also leads to weight gain, which is the exact opposite of your goal. According to the American Psychological Association, weight loss is never successful if you remain burdened by stress or other negative feelings. It's impossible to think stress won't occur during the 12-week program, or longer, if you have a significant amount of fat to lose. Stress can tip you in the wrong direction.

Since it is imperative to your success, you will need to learn how to cope with it.

Before we get into stress management, let's talk briefly about what happens in your body when you experience a stressor. Stress is a natural, physical, and mental reaction to good and bad experiences. When your body experiences a threat, or stress, it reacts with what is called a fight or flight response, which kicks in to protect your body acting as though your survival is on the line (see figure 6). The process starts in your brain. Your hypothalamus, located at the base of your brain, tells your adrenal glands, located atop the kidneys, to release adrenaline and cortisol.

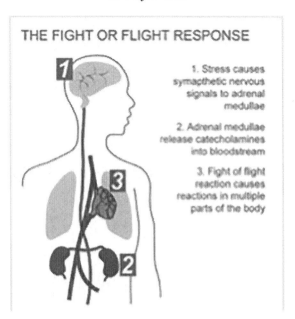

Figure 6. Fight or Flight Response (Source: "Fight or Flight Reaction." Haiku Deck: Presentation Software and Online Presentation Tools. Accessed December 2017. https://www.haikudeck.com/fight-or-flight-reaction-science-and-technology-presentation-jeQv1qWR8x#slide5.)

Adrenaline increases your heart rate, raises your blood pressure, and provides energy. Cortisol increases sugar in the blood stream by stimulating fat and carbohydrate metabolism to supply the body with fast energy. These stress hormones combined make blood vessels constrict and raises your blood pressure, which gets more oxygen to your brain and heart, so you have additional strength and energy. When these stress hormones are released, your liver produces extra blood sugar or glucose for additional energy. Blood flow to unnecessary organs or systems is also restricted, so more blood can flow to the muscle groups needed to assist with the flight or fight response.

Your heart rate increases allowing for more blood flow, and your digestion slows down. Even your pupils dilate to increase awareness of your surroundings. The body's response to stress is nothing short of AMAZING, especially when you consider this happens in seconds. The stress response is a good thing. After the threat has passed, the fight or flight is over, and the body systems return to their normal functions. However, if stress is chronic, and we don't turn off the stress response, we're in trouble. Every time we experience a stressor, even if it's not a life threatening stress, our body activates the stress response.

We don't want chronic stress, meaning our stress response system is turned on for a prolonged period, because it over-exposes us to stress hormones, which ultimately will wreak havoc on our body. Chronic stress negatively affects your overall health, physically, mentally, and emotionally. It affects every system in your body—your immune, endocrine, respiratory, cardiovascular, digestive, muscular, reproductive, and central nervous systems. It also compromises your brain function, leads to over or under eating, as well as alcohol and drug abuse.

Chronic stress affects us in many ways: increased appetite, high blood pressure, fatigue, depression, anxiety, weight gain, relationship problems, muscle pains, heart disease, infertility, digestive problems, memory and concentration problems, premature aging, headaches, hormone imbalances, difficulty sleeping, and Type 2 Diabetes or insulin resistance.

How does stress make you fat? Overgard conducted a study amongst a group of 6,704 nurses to test a theory that increased workload, and by association, higher levels of stress, contributed to an increased level of weight gain. He ultimately concluded that individuals who suffer from chronic stress may overeat to reduce the level of activity in the chronic stress response.[1]

Elevated cortisol levels increase the accumulation of abdominal fat, visceral fat. This is extremely harmful. This fat is different from subcutaneous fat cells in the rest of your body. Visceral fat contributes to cardiovascular disease, which is the number one killer of people worldwide, and diabetes, the fastest growing global disease.

---

1   Overgaard, D., M. Gamborg, F. Gyntelberg, and B. L. Heitmann. "Psychological workload is associated with weight gain between 1993 and 1999: analyses based on the Danish Nurse Cohort Study." *International Journal of Obesity* 28, no. 8 (2004): 1072-081. June 22, 2004. Accessed December 2017. doi:10.1038/sj.ijo.0802720

The movement of sugar (carbohydrates and fat metabolized) from our blood to our muscles requires insulin. High levels of sugar and insulin will cause your body to store fat. Scientists have discovered that fat cells actually have special receptors for the stress hormone cortisol. There are more of these receptors in our abdominal fat cells than anywhere else in our body. Also, high levels of cortisol negatively impact the way we respond to leptin. As we learned in a previous chapter, leptin is the hormone that tells us we're full. When that's not working properly, we tend to overeat.

We face many stressors in life: major life changes, traffic jams, negative life events, finances or money, family issues, poor nutrition, menopause, buying a house, getting married, getting divorced, death of a loved one, getting promoted, work deadlines, always staying connected, chronic worry, and a negative outlook. These are just a few. I'm sure you can add to this list. How do most people deal with stress? Typically, they compound the problem, ultimately creating more stress. They consume too much alcohol, eat comfort foods, which are usually high in sugar and simple carbohydrates, or they sit and watch television or their computer screen. All of these scream weight gain.

Enough about why stress is bad. You've experienced it, and you know how it can turn your world upside down. Let's talk about ways to manage stress so it doesn't interfere with our fat loss efforts. Exercise. Exercise is the number one way to manage stress. Besides burning calories, properly done exercise offsets the negative effects of the stress hormones, adrenaline and cortisol. It helps control sugar and insulin levels. The next best way to manage your stress is a healthy diet. As mentioned earlier, eating nutritious food throughout the day keeps blood levels stable and helps reduce insulin and cortisol levels. Another way to manage stress is getting proper sleep, seven to nine hours daily. When you deprive your body of sleep, cortisol levels rise, which results in feeling hungry. As discussed earlier, studies have shown a direct correlation between lack of sleep and simple carbohydrate intake, which causes insulin to rise.

You're probably thinking, if I follow *ThePerfectScale*, I'm already managing stress through nutrition, exercise, and sleep, so what's your point? In response, I say, "That's correct." Exercise, eating properly, and sleeping are great ways to manage your stress. However, there's one more stress management tool that I haven't discussed, and it's required for you to earn a point for stress management: relaxed breathing exercises or meditation, exercise for your brain. Meditation counters the biochemical effects of stress. It's almost the exact opposite of the stress response. It soothes your nervous system, allows you to get rid of agitation from stress, slows down your heart rate, and decreases your blood pressure. Meditation restores your body to a nice, calm state.

To meditate effectively, sit in a relaxed position, still your body, and clear your mind, essentially narrow your focus and shut out the external world. That's it. Stay there—sitting and breathing—for 10 to 15 minutes. Don't make this any harder than that. Distractions will come up, but just move them out of your mind and focus on breathing and relaxing. By doing this, you are simply clearing your mind and calming your body, which is needed in our 24/7/365 connected world. This simple, free activity has incredible benefits like improving your immune system, improving your memory, lowering your blood pressure, improving your physical and emotional response to stress, increasing your self-awareness, reducing your aging, giving you more energy, making you more productive, and improving your attention span. It also encourages a healthy lifestyle, improves your quality of sleep, increases your happiness, and strengthens your mind.

There are no negative side effects, and it's absolutely free. I can tell you that I've put people through this fat loss program that do not meditate. Although they had good results, they did not fare nearly as well as those who incorporated daily meditation. Learning to meditate will pay benefits for your entire life since you encounter stressors all the time. I have live(d) a stressful life, but I am taking measures to reduce and eliminate stress in my life because the truth is stress kills, and it is often self-imposed.

Between clients, teaching, running a business, children, and everything else in my life, I felt the need to slow down, relax, and meditate. At first, I thought I didn't have time. But I learned the importance of making time. I wish I had started meditating much earlier in my life because it has actually increased my productivity. For those of you who are doubting this part of the program, and I know there are some of you out there, I say simply just do it. You literally have nothing to lose. You waste 10 to 15 minutes several times a day watching TV, having meaningless conversations, surfing the web, or whatever your time-wasters may be.

Now I'll admit, I'm still a rookie at this, and by no means do I claim to be an expert in meditation. There is much more for me to learn, but you don't need to be an expert in order to get started and reap the benefits. There are two common styles of meditation: Mindfulness and Transcendental Meditation or TM. You can research them both to determine which works best for you. I can tell you that Hollywood is abuzz with TM. I chose the other type, mainly because it was inexpensive and required less time.

To get started, I suggest doing what I did. I went to Fragrantheart. com and clicked on their free link to learn how to meditate in five days. If you do this, every day, you will be sent a short meditation. The first meditation is two minutes. The next is four minutes, then six, eight, and then eventually 10 minutes. In five days, you will be meditating for 10 minutes. This is so easy, and it's the way to go. Warning, on the outset, I tried to sit down and meditate for 10 minutes, but it was painful and it felt like hours. I tried again and then I gave up. It wasn't until I found this program at Fragrantheart. com that I got on the right track. I strongly recommend it (I receive no compensation from the site. I just think it's a great resource, and it was very helpful to me.)

From there, I went to YouTube and reviewed hundreds of meditation videos. To this day, I catalog the ones I like, and I've created a library of 10 to 20 minute meditations. I share this in my courses and with my coaching clients.

Daily stress management counts for one point on the scale. While it counts for one point, it can play a much bigger role in your daily score, so don't ignore it. In order to get the point for stress management, you are required to meditate for 10 to 15 minutes. Ten minutes is the absolute minimum, and it must be done in one sitting.

I strongly recommend working your way up to 20 minutes. This can be done in one sitting for 20 minutes or two 10 minute sittings. I've found that with 20 minutes, I reaped significantly more benefits than 10 minutes. The additional 10 minutes was worth it as I felt better, my head and thoughts were clearer, my focus was pinpoint accurate, and I found myself much better equipped to handle stressful situations. All of which is supported by the research.

Meditation Tips:

- Take responsibility for your stress
- Find a quiet and private place to meditate
- Meditate sometime during the day if possible. In the morning, you are coming off a restful night's sleep and stress hasn't begun. At night, you're winding down and preparing to sleep. The time to quiet your mind and get focused is during the day when stressful events are constantly coming your way
- Try to meditate at the same time and place each day
- Use guided meditation that makes meditating simple. Just follow the guide
- Work on eliminating your stress. You may not be able to leave your job, change your commute, dissolve your marriage, or fix your finances overnight; however, you should put a plan in place to address any chronic stressor so that it is reduced and eventually eliminated
- Go to Fragrantheart.com and sign up for their "Learn to Meditate in 5 Days"

Chapter 13—The Negatives

You now should understand the 10 point scale and how you earn your points. Here's a quick review: Five points for meals, one point for exercise, one point for sleep, one point for hydration, one point for meditation, and one point for planning. Now let's talk about how you lose points. There are two ways to lose points: consuming alcohol and eating added sugar. Since alcohol and sugar are toxins, a poison, it will negatively affect your fat loss efforts. We'll address these issues separately. Let's start with alcohol.

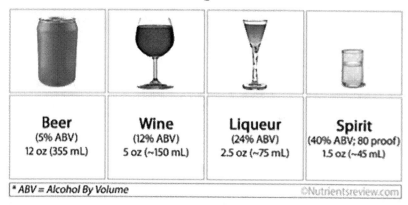

Figure 7. Amount of Alcohol in Standard Drinks (Source: Nutrients Review)

An alcoholic drink is five ounces of wine; one and a half ounces of an 80-proof liquor, vodka or whiskey for instance; or 12 ounces of beer. Alcohol is referred to as empty calories because while a gram is seven calories, it doesn't have any protein, carbohydrates, or fats. One of the problems with empty calories is they don't provide a feeling of satiety. Chances are you will consume alcoholic calories in addition to your food and end up overeating. In fact, research has shown that when alcohol is consumed before a meal, you eat 20 percent more calories. That number increases to 33 percent when you add the calories from the alcohol! Look at the list below of the caloric content of popular drinks.

Table 6. Calories in Popular Drinks

Type of Alcoholic Beverage	Approximate Calories
Regular Beer (12 fl.oz)	150
Light Beer (12 fl.oz)	105
Red Wine (5 fl.oz)	125
White Wine (5 fl.oz)	120
Champagne (4 fl.oz)	80
Martini (2.25 fl.oz)	124
Manhattan (2.25 fl.oz)	135
Cosmopolitan (2.75 fl.oz)	146
Mojito (6 fl.oz.)	143
Pina Colada (9 fl.oz)	490
Bloody Mary (4.6 fl.oz)	120
B-52 (1.5 fl.oz)	91
Screwdriver (7 fl.oz)	208
Margarita (4 fl.oz)	168
Rye, Rum, Vodka, Gin, Tequilla (1.5 fl.oz)	97

Source: Healthy Weight Loss Help

These drinks will cause you to go over your allotted calories for the day. That's a problem, but not the only problem with alcohol. The diagram below demonstrates the bigger problem with alcoholic consumption. Fat metabolism gets de-prioritized because your body makes breaking down alcohol the top priority. Since it's a toxin, it gets immediate attention. Unfortunately, your body can't store calories from alcohol and burn them later like it does food.

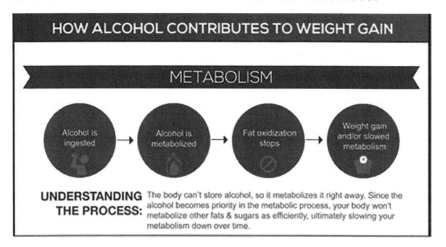

Figure 7. *How Alcohol Contributes to Weight Gain (Source: "Alcohol & Weight Gain." Lucas James | Celebrity Personal Trainer. November 07, 2014. Accessed December 2017. http://lucasjamespersonaltraining.com/ alcohol-weight-gain-infographic/4180/?utm_source=DesignTAXI&utm_ medium=DesignTAXI&utm_term=DesignTAXI&utm_ content=DesignTAXI&utm_campaign=DesignTAXI.)*

This means your metabolic system must stop what it's doing, which is burning fat, and start metabolizing the alcohol. Also, unlike food, alcohol needs no digestion. The calories from alcohol get used for energy instead of fat. Since your body can't break down carbohydrates and fat while processing alcohol, they get converted to body fat and move through your system for storage. Yes, storage spells fat gain. Can you say beer belly? Just think, when you consume alcohol, the fire alarm inside your body goes off and starts yelling, "Intruder! Intruder!" Everything stops and addresses the intruder. Whatever your body was doing, it's put on the back burner or should I say, your butt or gut? To summarize, the moment you consume alcohol your body works to eliminate it. This effort to eliminate it brings your metabolism or current fat burning to a halt. It must process the toxins first, which increases the risk that food that you've been consuming, will be stored as fat.

There are other disadvantages to alcohol consumption:

- It disrupts your sleep
- It releases estrogen into your bloodstream
- It's a diuretic. It may cause you to lose vital nutrients and minerals
- It promotes fat storage
- It will increase your cortisol levels
- It has no nutritional value, while containing seven calories per gram
- It may cause a decrease in testosterone in men
- It stimulates appetite
- It decrease motivation to exercise
- It ultimately will increase caloric intake

Even given the aforementioned, I still see a bigger problem with alcohol: It lowers your inhibitions!!! In a fat loss program, that's the last thing you need. That has "extra calories" written all over it, and that's not good. Guess what? Those extra calories are usually not healthy calories, not at all, not when alcohol is involved. Do you really think it's a good idea to impair your judgment and lower your inhibitions, which ends up stimulating your appetite on a fat loss program? Stay as far away from the booze as possible.

Unfortunately, the reality is that alcohol is part of the fabric of America, just like eating out. We like our alcohol, but it doesn't have a place in your fat loss program. Don't worry, I'm not recommending that you stop drinking for the rest of your life. That's not necessary. In fact, some alcohol consumption can be good for you. Once you're done with fat loss, I'll show you how to consume alcohol in the maintenance stage. In terms of *ThePerfectScale—The Ultimate Fat Loss System*, the moment alcohol hits your lips, you get a minus one; you lose a point for the day. If you drink two or more drinks, you get a minus two. If you consume one, high calorie or sugary drink, such as a Margarita, you receive a minus two. See the chart below for simple scoring on alcohol consumption.

Table 7. Negative Points for Consuming Alcohol

Number of Drinks	Women	Men
1 drink	-1	-1
2 drinks	-2	-1
More than 2	-2	-2

The negative impact for consuming alcohol is greater for women than men because on average, women weigh less than men resulting in less water in their bodies. Alcohol mostly resides in body water; therefore, the impact of an alcoholic beverage on blood alcohol concentration is greater for women.

Consuming more than two drinks will eliminate your chance of burning fat for the day, put you at risk of losing more points by over eating and not sleeping, and put you in danger of over eating the following day. These scores work if you drink once or twice a week. If you drink more than twice a week, unfortunately, the values increase on and after your 3rd drinking day. See chart two below. **If you are serious about losing fat, don't drink.** If you must, don't drink more than once or twice a week.

Table 8. Negative Points for Consuming Alcohol after 2 Days in a Week

Number of Drinks	Women	Men
1 drink	-2	-2
2 drinks	-3	-2
More than 2	-3	-3

I strongly recommend that you refrain from drinking alcohol while on this plan; however, that may be unrealistic for you. Considering holidays, work functions, social events, celebrations, and stress, there will be plenty of opportunities to indulge. In fact, 25 percent of our population drinks daily. I used to be part of that group. Fortunately, I addressed the stress and prioritized my goals, so I don't feel the need to drink daily. I have provided some tips below so that you know how to consume alcohol while on the program when a situation comes up.

Tips:

- Set a limit in terms of how many drinks you're going to consume before you start
- Alternate drinks with glasses of water
- Use low calorie mixers or lemon or lime
- Skip mixers and drink alcohol straight
- If you're out and ordering food, order your food before you order a drink
- Try to drink only on a high calorie day
- Don't have more than two drinks in one sitting
- Select wine or alcohol and use a zero-calorie mixer
- Have a wine spritzer instead of a glass of wine
- Don't skip a meal to conserve calories for drinking
- Don't drink sugary cocktails. Sorry, no margaritas until you're in maintenance mode. No craft beers either
- Drink after you finish your meal, if possible
- Don't consume snacks while you drink. Plan to skip the peanuts, pretzels, and chips

The other negative is sugar. Just like alcohol, added sugar is toxic to your body. Some organizations think it should be regulated like alcohol. We know sugar is everywhere. We enjoy it on holidays, at work functions, social events, celebrations, and whenever we want. It also is a stress reliever. Unfortunately, kids under the age of 21 can consume sugar and many parents unknowingly give it to their children in large quantities. Think the next time you give your child a soda, you just handed them a beer or a cigarette. It may seem a little unrealistic to you, but added sugar can eventually lead to heart disease, diabetes, obesity, cancer, and addiction, just like alcohol and cigarettes.

The problem with added sugars is that they are refined and concentrated. They overwhelm the body, which has a hard time storing and using them properly. Just like alcohol, when they are consumed, they set off a fire alarm. The average American eats approximately 120 to 160 pounds of added sugar per year! That's nearly three pounds a week, or a quarter to a half pound a day. This stuff is everywhere and can be difficult to avoid. Here's a quick list of so-called healthy food items with significant added sugar: bread, granola bars, yogurt, peanut butter, cereals, ketchup, fruit snacks, spaghetti sauce, almond milk, barbecue sauce, pretzels, graham crackers, and there are many more. The good thing is none are on our food list except natural peanut butter.

The recommended guideline is no more than 10 percent of your calories should come from added sugar. The World Health Organization recently lowered that to five percent. However, the average American consumes about 16 percent of their calories from added sugar. According to the University of California, Berkeley, the average American consumes 22 to 28 teaspoons of added sugar per day. No wonder diabetes is an epidemic.

What does five percent of your daily calories break down to? It equals six teaspoons of sugar for women, which is 24 grams or approximately 100 calories. For men, it means nine teaspoons of sugar, which is 36 grams or approximately 150 calories. It translates to three teaspoons of sugar for children, which is 12 grams or approximately 50 calories. When you eat added sugar, it basically gets converted and stored as fat. This occurs because when you consume large amounts of sugar, your liver must convert it to fat quickly. This fat moves around in your bloodstream where it can clog your arteries and be stored as fat on your butt or gut. Your body will use some of the converted sugar for energy, but this will cause it to stop burning fat, thus leading to additional storage.

Additionally, too much sugar causes your body to increase its insulin levels to get it out of the bloodstream and into your cells. This continued state of increased insulin in your body ultimately leads to your cells ignoring it. Your pancreas has no idea the insulin is being ignored, so it keeps producing it because you continue to consume the added sugars. Eventually your pancreas gets tired and stops working. Can you say hello to diabetes?

What are these added sugars? There are plenty of them. Anything on a label that ends in ose—sucrose, lactose, maltose, dextrose, fibose, linose, fructose, and galactacose—high fructose corn syrup, agave syrup, maple syrup, honey, table sugar, and molasses. The truth is this stuff really is addicting. Sugar stimulates the brain's reward pathway just like an opioid would. It is also habit forming. Like many drugs, you can acquire a tolerance to it, meaning it takes more and more to get stimulated. You eat more, you crave more. You can get caught in a vicious cycle just like a drug addict. The only difference is sugar isn't considered a drug, and it's everywhere and in almost everything.

Added sugar is used in approximately 75 percent of packaged foods. That's right, 75 percent. That's why when you look at the food list for this plan; you won't see packaged food items on it. These added sugars lead to a big spike in glucose followed by a big drop, leaving you hungry and wanting more. Your willpower is no match for this. You will find natural sugars on the list: whole fruits, vegetables, legumes, nuts, and some grains. Since the sugar in these items is consumed with water, fiber, and nutrients that are healthy to your body, it is released much more slowly into your body, and it provides constant energy. However, the biggest difference is they don't cause that huge spike that added sugars do instead they provide quality sugar that the body turns to glucose and uses for energy. While you want to steer clear of sugar, adding natural raw sugars, like honey or maple syrup, to your oatmeal, tea, or coffee is fine.

In terms of scoring on *ThePerfectScale—The Ultimate Fat Loss System*, any food or beverage you consume with added sugar, you receive a minus one. This includes a cookie, a small brownie, or any similar type food. If you consume a significant amount, then it would be a minus two. A significant amount would be a large piece of cake, an entire candy bar, or an entire soda. I know dark chocolate is good for you; however, it's not on the plan. You can enjoy that when you reach the maintenance stage.

Here are some tips to keep added sugars out of your fat loss plan.

- Avoid artificial sweeteners
- Use Stevia if you need to add a sweetener

- Never drink soda or energy drinks. Avoid eating cake, candy, cookies, pies, fruit drinks, or juices, ice cream, or anything similar
- Avoid flavored coffees
- Use table sugar in moderation. A teaspoon or two in your coffee is sufficient, no more
- Lastly, consume the foods on the list. Following the meal plan will keep you below the daily sugar consumption level recommended by the World Health Organization and American Heart Association. It will also keep your body in fat-burning mode

Chapter 14—Eating Out

According to the National Restaurant Association, there are over a million restaurants in America. The U.S. restaurant industry's food and drinks sales reached $700 billion in 2015, a long way from the $42.8 billion in 1970. In 2011, the average number of meals purchased at a restaurant within the United States was 194 per person. That's a lot of eating out. As we continue to eat out, we continue to grow larger and larger. Eating out has become the norm and, unfortunately, so is being overweight. When you eat out, you eat more because the portion sizes are larger. More food on the plate means more sales, and restaurants like sales (see figure 8).

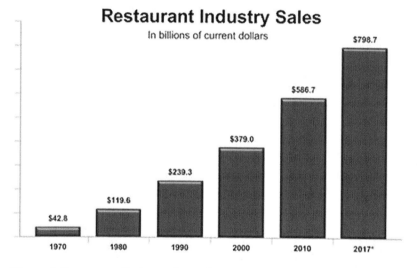

Figure 8. Restaurant Industry Sales. (Source: National Restaurant Association)

Eating out has contributed greatly to the obesity epidemic in our country. Americans spend as much money eating out as they do in grocery store purchases!!!

If people knew how to eat out to lose weight or maintain their weight, it wouldn't be as much of a problem. I must say I'm guilty of eating out. I love eating out. Why? The food tastes better in most cases, I don't have to clean up, and it's a great social environment. While I can cook, and I enjoy my cooking, I'm not nearly as good as the professionals. I can't create some of the dishes I like to eat when I go out. I like fine dining from time to time, and I love ethnic food. You probably eat out for similar reasons. However, when your goal is fat loss, you have to be careful when you eat out. If you don't know what you're doing, you're screwed. In this chapter, I'm going to teach you how to eat out while pursuing fat loss.

Now, remember the restaurant also has several goals:

1. Make money
2. Make sure that the food tastes good
3. Build the average check
4. Make sure you have a great experience
5. Get you to come back

How do they do this? First, they offer you drinks before you get your food. They loosen up your inhibitions first, and remember from last chapter, food always tastes good after alcohol. They offer you bread or something for free to add value. Next, they give you a generous, over-sized meal, so you perceive it as a great value. They add salt, sugar and extra fat so that it tastes delicious. That's why it tastes better when they cook it. Lastly, they offer you a sweet treat at the end to top it off, which leaves you with a smile and boosts the check. It's hard not to fall into this trap.

Before I delve into eating out for fat loss, I want you to know that any time you're eating whether at home or out, you fall into one of three categories. I mentioned them earlier in the book, but I will here again. You are either eating to gain fat/weight, eating to maintain fat/weight or eating to lose fat/ weight. That's it. It's one of the three. Most people think they're eating to maintain or lose weight when in fact they're eating to gain weight. If you've ever thought you were eating properly and wondered why you weren't losing weight, chances are this was your problem. Let me explain each category in reference to eating out.

EATING TO GAIN FAT/WEIGHT

While eating out, these people use words like, "Yes, please, and thank you." When they go out, they have no advance plan on what to eat, and they end up eating whatever sounds good or looks good on the menu. Since they have no idea the menu was designed to fatten them up and accomplish the restaurant's goals, the restaurant takes control of them. They think they're making the choice, but they often end up saying, "Yes, please or thank you" to the recommendations from the server.

For example, "Would you like some bread?"

"Yes."

"Would you like to hear about our specials?"

"Yes."

"Would you like another drink?"

"Thank you."

"We have some great desserts. Would you like to hear them?"

"Please."

When you're in this category, you often overeat. You can almost eat a day's worth of calories in one sitting. Let's take a look. Let's say at the start of the meal you have two drinks. That's anywhere between 200 to 300 calories. (That's for two glasses of wine. It's easy to consume more calories than this depending upon what you're drinking.) Next comes the bread and the dipping oil, another 200 to 300 calories. Then maybe an appetizer or salad. That can range anywhere between 200 to 300 calories, and that's a healthy salad with balsamic dressing. If you order onion rings or calamari, you'll easily consume more calories.

Then comes the entrée, which can be 500 to 700 calories (I'm being nice 700-1,000 calories is more likely). This will vary, but most people aren't ordering grilled chicken and steamed veggies when they go out. Then to top it off, you order the dessert, another 200 to 300 calories. I love cheesecake, and that's 400 calories before the topping. You can see when you add this up, it is anywhere between 1,300 to 1,800 or more calories, which is too many for one sitting, possibly too many for one day. And ALL of my estimates are on the low side. Keep in mind that it's very easy to justify consuming this; especially if you are drinking and you've been exercising. Recognize though, this has no place on a fat loss plan.

EATING TO MAINTAIN FAT/WEIGHT

If you're eating to maintain your weight, you have control. Remember this, because after you have completed *The Perfect Scale—The Ultimate Fat Loss System*, this is how you want to eat when you go out. The key phrase for this group is "choose your poison." Pick a "poison" and enjoy it. This gives you a plan and puts you in total control. When I say "choose a poison," I mean choose to have an appetizer and a healthy meal; or choose to have drinks, two or three, with a healthy meal; or choose to have a healthy meal and a dessert; or choose to have a meal that is not the healthiest, such as one higher in calories. You get one bad thing to enjoy.

What's a healthy meal? Protein with a salad and/or a veggie. You can also eat good quality grains, although they may not be on the menu. Just be careful because they may be cooked for taste and, therefore, full of salt and fat. Portion control is key to maintenance, so make sure you don't overeat. Take home the leftovers. For me, when I eat out, my poison is alcohol. I'll eat a healthy meal, skip the bread, appetizer, and dessert, and if I'm going for it, I'll have a third drink. I try to stop at three, or it may turn into a late-night burger binge. When that happens, I'm no longer eating to maintain instead I'm eating to gain fat/weight.

EATING TO LOSE FAT/WEIGHT

If you're eating to lose fat/weight, then learn to use the phrase, "No, thank you." Remember, you're in total control of your answers to questions from the bartender and wait staff. You simply say, "No, thank you."

"Would you like a drink?"

"No, thank you."

"Would you like bread?"

"No, thank you."

"Would you like to see the dessert menu?"

"No, thank you."

When I'm in this mode, I don't even want to see the menu. I've predetermined my dinner before I have even gone out, and I don't order any drinks. I just order some seltzer or water with a lemon or lime so I have something in my hand if I get thirsty. Steer clear of the alcohol.

What does a fat loss meal look like in a restaurant? It looks the same way it does on your meal plan: protein and double vegetables or protein, salad, and a vegetable. I recommend you stay away from the grains unless you know for sure it's been prepared in a healthy manner.

Feel free to order something not listed specifically on their menu. Anything you see on the menu is available in a healthy option. If you see Chicken Parmesan, then they have grilled chicken or seared chicken. If you want to splurge when you're eating for fat loss, order a healthy appetizer, shrimp cocktail or a salad. Don't let eating out ruin your daily score. When you're on the plan, try not to eat out often, and leave soon after you've finished eating. This keeps the temptation to a minimum.

Here are some tips.

- Drink two glasses of water before you eat
- Eat throughout the day. Follow your usual meal plan, and then eat according to your meal plan at the restaurant
- Review the menu ahead of time. Go online, browse the menu, and decide what you're going to eat before you go. You can't go wrong with a protein and two servings of vegetables and a salad

- Remember you don't have to order from the menu. Think . . . If it's a burger joint, it doesn't have to come with a bun. Get the burger on top of a salad and skip the fries
- Always, always, always pass on the bread. It's just not worth it

TWO FINAL NOTES ON EATING OUT

1. Make sure if you go off the plan that it's worth it. Ask yourself, "Is this worth it?" If the answer is yes, then do it, but be reasonable. If you're going off your plan, remember to choose your poison. You can't have it all. Cocktails, bread, appetizer, a high calorie meal, and dessert is pure gluttony. Just pick your poison, choose one, only one, and enjoy. Pass on the appetizer unless it's healthy like a shrimp cocktail. Do not order a meal with gluten or dairy. Remember, I will explain how you consume those in the maintenance stage. They have no business on a weight loss plan.

2. Be careful about the portion size. There's nothing wrong with leftovers. Don't overeat. If you don't overeat, you can't gain weight. Don't let sugar ruin your meal. If you have to eat dessert, don't eat dessert alone. Share it. Spread the poison around. If you're going to drink, don't drink heavy drinks or fruity drinks and make sure you watch the mixers. Club soda is a good mixer. Enjoy fresh fruit like lemons and limes.

Chapter 15—Action

Let's start with a quick review of how to use *ThePerfectScale—The Ultimate Fat Loss System* properly.

Nutrition—you earn one point for each of the required five daily meals that follows the nutrition guidelines of your meal plan. Thus, that's five points a day.

Exercise/Rest—you earn one point per day for exercising or resting, and you're expected to exercise five days a week, and rest two days.

Hydration—you can earn one point a day by drinking half your body weight in ounces of water. If, for example, you weigh two hundred pounds, you need to drink one hundred ounces of water daily.

Sleep—you earn one point if you sleep for seven to nine hours a night.

Stress Management—you earn a point if you meditate each day for 10-15 minutes.

Planning—you earn one point for planning for the following day, including packing any meals that you will not be eating at home, knowing what you're ordering if you eat out, knowing your workout time, having workout clothes ready, knowing when and where stress management will take place, and knowing what's for dinner the following day. (Planning is done the night before)

Now, you don't have to get a 100 percent, 10 points, every day. If you can get 10 out of 10 points every day for twelve weeks, that's phenomenal. You will turn back the clock 10 years! Not everyone, however, can be the valedictorian of the class. Your goal should be ten points, but you will experience fat loss with a nine, or eight points, as well. The most important part of *ThePerfectScale—The Ultimate Fat Loss System*, besides the score is the immediate feedback. Use it as a tool to fix a problem you've identified. If you keep getting four out of five points on nutrition, then focus on your food, identity the problem, and institute changes to fix it. The same thing with sleep. If you can't get seven hours of sleep on a regular basis, figure out what's preventing you from sleeping and address it. This is why *ThePerfectScale* is truly the only scale for fat loss.

It not only gives you a daily grade, but it identifies areas where you can improve. Again, your goal is 10 points; however, eight or nine points will allow you to continue to be in a fat loss mode, but you just won't lose fat as fast. Seven or eight points, and you're in maintenance. Drop below seven, and you're in weight gain. Now you have the information you need to pursue long term fat loss. I've made fat loss as simple as possible for you. Is more information necessary? No. The key now is to put what you know into action and get started.

There is one more piece of advice, however, that is imperative to your success. Think back to anything you've achieved, either personally or professionally. From college degrees, to raising children, to purchasing a home, anything. Anything that you're proud of or have accomplished. Three things were involved, and every success story contains these three elements: focus, discipline, and consistency. It's impossible to have any degree of success in anything without them, especially fat loss and lifestyle change. Let's examine these three words a little further.

Focus–a point of concentration. If you're going to make significant changes to your body, it's going to take time, at least three months and more if you have a significant amount of weight to lose. A clear focus, a mental picture of exactly what you want to accomplish, will allow you to stay the course. If you lose your focus, you won't make it to your goal instead you will become distracted by the "things" that will knock you off course and cloud your vision. With a clear focus, "things" may attempt to creep in, but you won't allow them to ruin your plan. You will figure out a way to handle whatever comes up, while staying focused on your goals.

Discipline–the training to act in accordance with established rules. As you know, part of losing fat is eating healthy, exercising, hydrating, resting, managing stress, and planning. Here is where discipline comes into play. Eating healthy is easy to say, but hard to do in the fast paced, fast food, unhealthy environment in which we live. Exercising for fat loss requires hard work; you need to do more than walk on the treadmill, or spend a half hour on the elliptical. You need to put yourself in an uncomfortable state in order to create a metabolic disturbance, which will allow you to boost your metabolism and burn fat. You will need discipline to say "No" frequently to all the things that can sneak in and make you lose your focus. When everyone wants pizza and beer, you need to be disciplined. When you are tempted to over indulge in wine, you need to be disciplined. Going to the gym after a hard day at work instead of going home requires discipline.

Consistency–steadfast adherence to the same principles. Consistency is good habits over a lengthy period of time. One great day of eating and exercising will do nothing; one week will make you feel a little better; one month will create a habit that will lead to major visual changes if you remain consistent and continue for another month or two. The consistent application of healthy eating, exercising, hydrating, resting, meditating, and planning will allow you to lose fat, live a healthy lifestyle, and turn the clock back 10 years.

Before you think about how you're going to change your eating, or how many times you're going to get to the gym, answer the important questions:

- What do you really want to accomplish?
- What's your short and long term goal?
- What sacrifices are you willing to make to get there? What are you willing to give up?
- What are you going to eliminate or change in your life so that you can behave in a disciplined manner?
- How is your schedule going to change so you can exercise consistently?
- How and when are you going to prepare meals?

These are just some of the questions that you should ask before you get started. You should only get started after you've answered these questions.

If you need further support and knowledge to get through this program, go to my website, TheFitnessProfessor.com. I have a ton of resources there for you. Yes, some require a fee, but I can promise you two things. First, the value you will receive will be worth much more than what you pay. Second, if you're not successful, I'll give you your money back. I have guarantees on all of my services. Think of it this way: You can learn how to drive by reading a book, or you can learn how to drive by getting behind the wheel, or you can learn how to drive by taking a course with a coach or a professional who is there to teach and mentor you along the way. Which of these choices do you think will give you the best success? I can put only so much information in the book, and I reserve plenty of information for my self-paced course and *ThePerfectScale Academy*. Participants in these courses are paying for a higher level of understanding. Not only do they get that, but they get access to information that's not readily available. Very few absorb everything in one reading. It takes time, action, and continued learning. If you're serious about losing fat and getting to maintenance, read the book again and make an investment in your health by registering for some of the other services I offer.

Figure 9 and 10 show my transformation after completing the program. Not bad for a 50 year old guy. My average daily score was slightly below 9. Which is proof that you don't have to be perfect, and you can turn the clock back 10 years in 12 weeks. I did go off meal plan and consume alcohol during the 12 weeks. You can see others on my website, TheFitnessProfessor.com

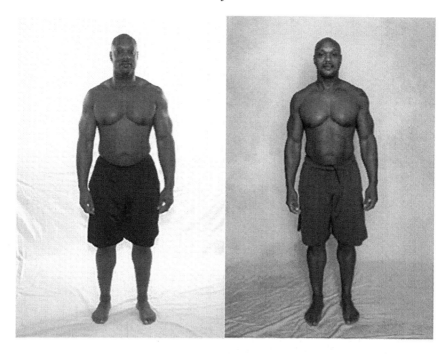

Figure 9. My transformation before and after the program: front view

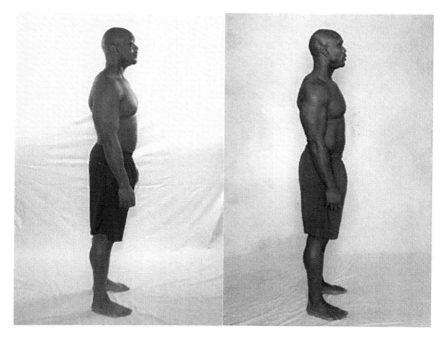

Figure 10. My transformation after the program: side view

WHAT'S NEXT?

If, after twelve weeks, you are not where you want to be, that's not a problem. You're on your way, and you will get there. However, you need to adjust your eating so your metabolism doesn't adjust to the reduction in calories. I recommend you increase your calories to a maintenance level for at least one to three months, and then go back to the fat loss program for another twelve weeks.

If you are still not where you want to be, repeat this process again: maintenance and then back to fat loss. This method will allow you to have the most success.

If you have achieved your desired goal, congratulations! You need to continue for one more month before going to the maintenance plan. Why? I recommend that you give yourself a little cushion so that you don't have to go back to the fat loss program. This extra month will allow you to continue to burn fat, and provide a cushion, so if for some reason you do put on a few pounds during maintenance, it's not a problem.

Maintenance means maintenance, so you shouldn't gain any weight during this phase, if you follow the guidelines in this book and score at least an 8 every day.

If you want to learn how to bring back the items we eliminated during the Fat lass program and exercise for maintenance you'll need to buy my next book, *Unscaled—How to Eat, Drink, and Be Merry Without Gaining Weight*. It should be on the shelves in April 2018.

I wish you nothing but the best in health and in life. Please keep in touch and send me your results and feedback to Feedback@ TheFitnessProfessor.com.

About the Author

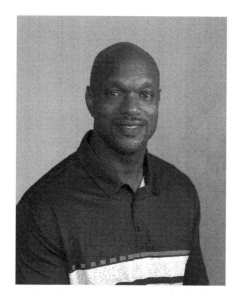

Doug Dorsey is a college professor, fitness coach, author, entrepreneur and healthy lifestyle transformation expert. With over two decades of college teaching experience and over a decade of personal training experience, Doug is one of the top personal fitness coaches around. Known as the Fitness Professor because of his educational approach to fitness, Doug employs a systematic approach to fat loss. Many of his ideas and philosophies are cutting edge, down to earth, and life changing.

Since it is his mission to help others improve their life through education and fitness, he lectures and speaks at corporate offices, businesses, and organizations looking to take a healthy and realistic approach to health and weight loss. Doug resides in West Hartford, Connecticut with his two beautiful daughters.

Made in the USA
Middletown, DE
02 September 2018